NOTES ON MEDICAL VIROLOGY

BY

MORAG C. TIMBURY

M.D., Ph.D., M.R.C.P.(Glasg.), M.R.C.Path.

Senior Lecturer in Virology,
University of Glasgow

Honorary Consultant Virologist,
Western Infirmary, Glasgow

FOREWORD

BY

J. H. SUBAK-SHARPE

B.Sc., Ph.D.

Professor of Virology, University of Glasgow

FOURTH EDITION

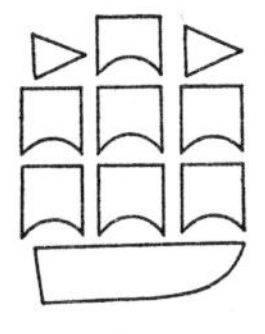

CHURCHILL LIVINGSTONE

EDINBURGH AND LONDON 1973

ISBN 0 443 00961 9

First edition . . .	1967
Second edition . . .	1969
Third edition . . .	1971
Fourth edition . . .	1973

Printed in Great Britain

NOTES ON MEDICAL VIROLOGY

FOREWORD

VIROLOGY concerns itself with viruses at many different levels—from the study at the molecular level of the structure, genetic information, content and function of the particle and the virus-host cell complex, via the analysis of the events which define the progress of viral disease in the host organism to interrelationships between the virus and populations of potential host organisms. These different levels necessarily have led to a dichotomy of virology into the pure and the applied field and, until now, medicine for all practical purposes has been almost solely concerned with the latter. But, as our knowledge of viruses at all analytical levels is becoming more and more extensive, and particularly if one considers the recent dramatic increase of our understanding of events at the molecular level, some knowledge of the general field of pure virology is bound to become relevant even for the doctor in general practice whose sole concern in the past has been with the field of applied virology. These notes are starting to bridge this gap.

Dr Timbury's lucid, concise and astonishingly comprehensive book of notes is particularly well suited to help medical students, who are primarily concerned with the spectrum of diseases caused by viruses, to get acquainted with the subject of virology. The book neither aims nor pretends to be a self-sufficient textbook, and, to this end, recommended references for further reading have been included. Clearly presented, informative and inexpensive, this book should prove most useful to students in conjunction with their course of lectures, practicals and hospital instruction.

The book, which is an excellent summary of the major virological problems in medicine, can be highly recommended for students of medicine.

J. H. SUBAK-SHARPE.

Glasgow, 1973.

PREFACE TO FOURTH EDITION

THIS book attempts to give a concise and factual account of medical virology. It is based on the lecture course given to medical students at the University of Glasgow who attend classes in the Western Infirmary. It is intended to be an accompaniment to lectures and should be supplemented by reading from one of the larger text books on virology. References to relevant articles and books have been included at the end of each chapter.

Viruses have been grouped primarily on the basis of the diseases which they cause. The clinical features and epidemiology of the diseases are described together with the characteristics of the viruses concerned, methods of laboratory diagnosis and details of the viral vaccines in current use. In addition to viruses which are important in medicine, tumour viruses are discussed because of their general interest and importance in biology. For this edition, a chapter on the biology of virus replication has been added. Rickettsiae and bedsonia are included because, although not true viruses, by tradition they are usually dealt with by virologists.

I should like to thank Professor J. H. Subak-Sharpe for writing the foreword and Professor N. R. Grist whose enthusiasm for virology was first responsible for my interest in the subject. I am grateful to Dr. Eleanor J. Bell and to Dr. T. H. Pennington for their advice on many points and for much helpful discussion. Thanks are also due to Mr. R. Callander, Department of Medical Illustration, University of Glasgow, who prepared the drawings and diagrams, and to Dr. E. A. C. Follett, Medical Research Council Virology Unit, Institute of Virology, Glasgow, who provided the electron micrograph of influenza virus particles which is reproduced on the cover.

MORAG C. TIMBURY

Glasgow, 1973.

CONTENTS

CHAPTER I

GENERAL PROPERTIES OF VIRUSES

VIRUSES are the smallest known infective agents. Most forms of life—animals, plants and bacteria—are susceptible to infection with appropriate viruses.

Three main properties distinguish viruses from other micro-organisms:—

1. *Small size*: Viruses are smaller than other organisms and vary in size from 10 nm to 300 nm. In contrast, bacteria are approximately 1,000 nm and erythrocytes are 7,500 nm in diameter.
2. *Genome*: The genome of viruses may be either DNA or RNA: most viruses contain only one type of nucleic acid but some RNA tumour viruses also possess a small piece of DNA.
3. *Metabolically inert*: Viruses have no metabolic activity outside susceptible host cells; they do not possess any ribosomes or protein-synthesising apparatus although some of the larger viruses contain one or more enzymes within their particles: viruses cannot therefore multiply in inanimate media but only inside living cells: on entry into a susceptible cell, however, the virus genome or nucleic acid is capable of replicating new virus particles.

STRUCTURE OF VIRUSES

Viruses consist basically of a core of nucleic acid surrounded by a protein coat.

The protein coat is antigenic and specific for each virus type: it protects the viral genome from inactivation by adverse environmental factors *e.g.* nucleases in the blood stream.

The structures which make up a virus particle are known as:—

virion—the intact virus particle
capsid—the protein coat
capsomeres—the protein sub-units of which the capsid is composed.
nucleic acid

envelope: the particles of many viruses are surrounded by a lipo-protein envelope usually partially derived from the outer membrane of the host cell.

Virus particles show three types of symmetry:—

Cubic— in which the particles are icosahedral protein shells with the nucleic acid contained inside

Helical—in which the particle is elongated and wound in the form of a helix or spiral: the capsomeres are arranged round the spiral of nucleic acid: most helical viruses possess an outer envelope

Complex—in which the particle does not conform to either cubical or helical symmetry.

CLASSIFICATION

There is as yet no entirely satisfactory classification of viruses: viruses are assigned to groups mainly on the basis of their nucleic acid and the symmetry and morphology of the virus particle.

The main groups of medically-important viruses together with some of their properties are shown in Table I.

TABLE I VIRUS GROUPS AND PARTICLES

GROUP	VIRUSES	PARTICLE
DNA viruses Poxviruses	variola, vaccinia, cowpox, alastrim, molluscum contagiosum, orf	large brick-shaped or oval virus particles with complex symmetry
Adenoviruses	adenoviruses	icosahedral particles with fibres projecting from apices
Herpesviruses	herpes simplex varicella-zoster cytomegalovirus E B virus	icosahedral particles surrounded by a loose envelope
Papovaviruses	papilloma polyoma, SV_{40}, virus of progressive multifocal leuco-encephalopathy	small icosahedral particles
RNA viruses Myxoviruses	influenza	enveloped roughly spherical particles with helical symmetry
Paramyxoviruses	parainfluenza, mumps, measles	enveloped roughly spherical particles with helical symmetry
Rhabdoviruses	rabies virus Marburg virus	bullet-shaped virus particles with envelopes: helical symmetry
Picornaviruses	enteroviruses rhinoviruses	small icosahedral particles
Reoviruses	reoviruses	medium sized icosahedral particles with double-shelled capsid
Togaviruses	yellow fever viruses of encephalitis, dengue, haemorrhagic fevers	enveloped particles with icosahedral symmetry
Arenoviruses	lymphocytic choriomeningitis virus: Lassa virus	round enveloped particles with internal granules

CULTIVATION OF VIRUSES

Since viruses will only replicate within living cells special methods have to be employed for culture *in vitro*: three main systems are used for cultivation of viruses in the laboratory.

1. **Tissue culture.** Cells obtained from man or animals are grown in artificial culture in glass vessels in the laboratory: these cells are living and metabolising and so can support viral replication: most—but not all—viruses can be propagated in cultures of suitable cells.
2. **Chick embryo.** Some viruses can be grown in the cells of the chick embryo: fertile eggs are kept in an incubator in the laboratory for this purpose: this technique has been largely superseded by tissue culture.
3. **Laboratory animals.** Before other techniques were available, viruses were isolated and studied mainly by inoculation of laboratory animals such as mice, rabbits, ferrets and monkeys: animals are still required for the isolation of some viruses.

EFFECTS OF VIRUSES ON CELLS

Viruses may affect cells in four main ways:—

Cell death. The infection is lethal and kills the cell—cytopathic effect (CPE).

Cell transformation. The cell is not killed but is changed in its properties *e.g.* from a normal cell to one with the properties of a malignant or cancerous cell.

Latent infection. The virus remains within the cell in a potentially active state but produces no obvious effect on the cell's functions.

HAEMAGGLUTINATION

Although viruses cannot grow in erythrocytes, many viruses cause erythrocytes to haemagglutinate or adhere together in clumps.

THE EFFECT OF PHYSICAL AND CHEMICAL AGENTS ON VIRUSES

HEAT: Most are inactivated at 56°C. for 30 minutes or at 100°C. for a few seconds: some are more resistant to heat.

COLD: Stable at low temperatures, most can be stored at −40°C. or, preferably, at −70°C.: some viruses are partially inactivated by the process of freezing and thawing.

DRYING: Variable. Some survive well, others are rapidly inactivated.

ULTRA-VIOLET IRRADIATION: Inactivates viruses.

CHLOROFORM AND ETHER: Viruses containing lipid are inactivated, those without lipid are resistant. Used for classification of viruses.

OXIDISING AGENTS: Viruses are inactivated by formaldehyde, chlorine, iodine and hydrogen peroxide.

PHENOLS: Most viruses are relatively resistant.

GLYCEROL: Viruses are resistant to glycerol which is therefore sometimes used as a preservative to prevent bacterial contamination of viral suspensions.

VIRUS DISEASES

Viruses are important and common causes of human disease especially in children: most viral infections are mild and the patient makes a complete recovery: many infections are in fact silent and the virus multiplies in the body without causing symptoms of disease: however, viral infections which are usually mild may occasionally cause severe disease in an unusually susceptible patient: a few viral diseases are severe and have a high mortality rate.

Entry: Viruses most often enter the body via the respiratory tract by inhalation but some viruses gain entry by ingestion or by inoculation through skin abrasions.

Virus diseases can be of two types:—

1. *Systemic*: the virus spreads widely and invades many tissues and organs—usually as a result of viraemia or virus in the blood stream: there is a relatively long incubation period *e.g.* childhood fevers such as measles and varicella.
2. *Localised*: the virus invades only tissues adjacent to the site of entry: the incubation period is usually short: most respiratory virus infections are of this type.

Invasiveness: virus disease is produced by direct spread of the virus to tissues and organs and not to toxin production as is the case in bacteria: the process of virus replication in the cells of the tissues usually—although not always—kills the infected cells: this may result in lesions and disease in the tissue concerned.

Non-specific defence mechanism of the host: the main defence mechanism of the body during the acute phase of virus infection is the production of a protein *interferon*: interferon is released from infected cells and, when taken up by other cells, renders them refractory to virus infection (see p. 111).

Immunity: virus infections are usually followed by immunity or resistance to re-infection with the same virus:

this is due to the appearance in the patient's serum of antibodies which neutralise the infectivity of the virus: neutralising antibodies generally persist for many years and prevent reinfection with the same virus: antibodies which fix complement are also produced but do not persist for so long as neutralising antibodies. Viral antibodies are found in the following immunoglobulins:—

IgM: 19S macroglobulins: present in serum: the earliest antibodies formed but persist for only a few weeks.

IgG: 7S globulins: also present in serum: appear later than IgM antibodies but persist for long periods of time—often for many years.

IgA: 7S-18S globulins: found in respiratory, salivary, intestinal or breast secretions: the most important antibody in immunity to respiratory virus diseases.

Further Reading

FENNER, F. (1968). *The Biology of Animal Viruses,* vol. 1, Molecular and Cellular Biology. New York: Academic Press.

CHAPTER II

THE BIOLOGY OF VIRUS REPLICATION

VIRUSES show a high degree of parasitism in that they are metabolically inert until they infect a susceptible cell: after invading a cell, viruses redirect the biochemical machinery of the cell to produce components for new virus particles: this is done by means of virus messenger RNA.

Production of virus messenger RNA is the most important function of the virus and is the basic mechanism which enables a virus to take over the functions of a cell.

Transcription: virus messenger RNA is made using the virus genome or nucleic acid as template: in this way, information which codes for virus proteins is passed from the virus genome via virus messenger RNA to the cell ribosomes where the proteins are synthesised.

Translation: virus messenger RNA attaches to the ribosomes and directs the formation of virus-specified proteins.

Virus-specified proteins are of two types:—

1. *Structural proteins*: which make up the capsids of new virus particles.
2. *Non-structural proteins*: which are not incorporated into new particles: many of these are enzymes required for the processes of virus replication—and especially for the synthesis of new virus nucleic acid molecules.

The number of proteins for which a virus can code is limited by the size of the virus genome.

Large viruses usually have high molecular weight nucleic acid: they can therefore code for many of the enzymes involved in their replication.

Small viruses have low molecular weight nucleic acid: they can code for very few proteins in addition to their structural proteins: because of this they may have to use some of the host cell's enzymes for their replication.
Cistrons: from the point of view of genetic functions, the virus genome can be sub-divided into cistrons each of which contains the information for the production of one functional polypeptide or protein.
Table II gives examples of the main virus groups with details about some properties of their genome.

VIRUS GROWTH CYCLE
INITIAL INTERACTIONS BETWEEN VIRUS AND CELL

The early part of the virus growth cycle can be divided into three stages:—

1. *Adsorption*: the first step in the invasion of a cell by virus: some—possibly all—viruses adsorb to specific receptors on the cell plasma membrane: viruses adsorb best at 37° but they also adsorb well although more slowly at 4° C.: divalent cations—Mg^{++} or Ca^{++}—enhance adsorption.
2. *Entry*: after adsorption, the cell membrane invaginates round the adsorbed virus particle: the virus is then engulfed by the cell within a pinocytotic vacuole: this process is temperature-dependent and takes place at 37° C. but not at 4° C.
3. *Uncoating*: the protein coat of the virus is removed: this is probably carried out by host cell enzymes contained in lysosomes: virus nucleic acid is then released or at least made accessible for the production of virus

TABLE II. SOME PROPERTIES OF VIRUS GENOMES

Virus	Nucleic acid			Transcriptase* contained in virus particles	Number of known virus structural proteins
	Type	Molecular weight ($\times 10^6$ daltons)	Infectivity		
Vaccinia	Double-stranded DNA	160	0	+	17
Herpes simplex	Double-stranded DNA	100	0	0	24
Adenovirus	Double-stranded DNA	23	+	0	5
Polyoma	Double-stranded DNA	3	+	0	6†
Poliovirus	Single-stranded RNA	2·6	+	0	4
Sindbis (a Togavirus)	Single-stranded RNA	3·5	+	0	3
Influenza A	Single-stranded RNA	2·8 - 4·0	0	+	7
Rous sarcoma	Single-stranded RNA	10	0	+	7

*DNA- or RNA-dependent RNA polymerase for synthesis of messenger RNA
†Three of these are host cell proteins and not virus-specified
Modified and reproduced, with permission, from a table originally drawn up by Dr. C. R. Pringle

messenger RNA: in the case of vaccinia virus a host cell enzyme removes the outer coat of the virus but a newly-made protein—which is probably virus-specified —carries out the final stripping of the particle.

BIOCHEMISTRY OF VIRUS REPLICATION

There are clearly basic differences in the biochemistry of the replication of DNA and RNA viruses: but in both cases, the fundamental purpose of the replicative process is the synthesis of:—

1. nucleic acid molecules
2. protein capsids

—which later become assembled into new, complete, infectious particles.

(i) DNA viruses

Nucleic acid: most DNA virus contain double-stranded DNA.

Virus messenger RNA: two types are produced:—

i. *early* messenger RNA: which codes mainly for the enzymes required for virus DNA synthesis.
ii. *late* messenger RNA: which is made after virus DNA synthesis and which codes mainly for virus structural proteins.

Transcription: with some DNA viruses, for example, herpes simplex and adenoviruses, early messenger RNA is replicated by host cell DNA-dependent RNA polymerase: in the case of vaccinia virus, the infecting virus particle contains a RNA polymerase with which early messenger RNA is transcribed.

Synthesis of progeny virus DNA molecules: in addition to the synthesis of virus proteins, an essential step in virus replication is the manufacture of DNA molecules for incorporation into new virus particles: many enzymes are involved in DNA synthesis but the most important is *DNA-dependent DNA polymerase*: uninfected host cells contain this enzyme and adenovirus seems to use the host cell enzyme for virus DNA replication: on the other hand herpes simplex and vaccinia viruses code for new virus-specified enzymes: these two viruses also code for some of the other enzymes required for DNA synthesis—for example, deoxythymidine kinase: DNA replication takes place early in the growth cycle before the synthesis of most structural proteins: the input strand of virus DNA acts as template for the production of progeny DNA molecules.

Late messenger RNA: is transcribed off progeny DNA molecules.

Virus structural proteins: are usually synthesised from late messenger RNA, that is, after virus DNA synthesis has taken place: however some vaccinia structural proteins are produced from early messenger RNA: vaccinia and herpes simplex viruses have a coat or envelope and a proportion of their structural proteins are carbohydrate-containing glycoproteins which form part of the outer covering of the virus particle: virus proteins are made in the cytoplasm and, as far as is known, synthesis is carried out using host cell transfer RNA species to transport amino acids to the ribosomes for incorporation into the developing polypeptide chain.

Site of replication: vaccinia virus replicates and is assembled entirely in the cytoplasm: the proteins of herpes simplex and adenoviruses are made in the cytoplasm but are transported to the nucleus for assembly into nucleocapsids or non-enveloped particles: herpes simplex later acquires an envelope by budding through the nuclear membrane of the cell.

(ii) **RNA viruses**

RNA viruses are unique in biology because their genetic material is contained in RNA instead of DNA: like DNA viruses, the crucial factor in infecting a cell is the production of virus messenger RNA: RNA viruses can be divided into two groups depending on the way in which their messenger RNA is formed:—

i. RNA viruses of which *the input strand of RNA in the infecting particle acts as messenger RNA*: the RNA of these viruses is infectious when extracted from virus particles and applied to cells.

ii. RNA viruses in which *the messenger RNA is transcribed off—and is therefore complementary to—the input strand of RNA*: particles of the viruses in this group contain a RNA polymerase which synthesises messenger RNA: RNA extracted from particles lacks this transcriptase and is therefore non-infectious.

Synthesis of progeny virus RNA molecules: most RNA viruses contain single-stranded RNA: the first step in virus RNA synthesis is the formation of a double-stranded RNA molecule called the replicative form: this is made by the synthesis of a strand of RNA which is complementary to the input strand and which remains associated with it: progeny RNA molecules are then made using the second or complementary strand of RNA as template: this stage is carried out by a virus-specified RNA-dependent RNA polymerase.

REPLICATION OF RNA VIRUSES OF WHICH THE INPUT STRAND FUNCTIONS AS MESSENGER RNA

The main example of this type of RNA virus is poliovirus.

Messenger RNA: after uncoating, the input strand of RNA

attaches to the host cell ribosomes and is translated into virus-specified proteins: these include virus structural proteins and non-structural proteins such as the enzyme RNA-dependent RNA polymerase which is required for the synthesis of virus RNA: this enzyme is not present in uninfected cells and must therefore be coded for by the virus genome.

Progeny virus RNA molecules: are replicated by the virus-coded RNA polymerase as described above; they have three different functions in the replicative cycle:

1. Templates for replicative forms for further virus RNA synthesis.
2. Genomes for newly-formed virus particles.
3. Virus messenger RNA molecules.

Virus proteins: poliovirus messenger RNA is multicistronic: this means that instead of coding for a series of separate polypeptides or proteins, the messenger RNA codes for a single very large polypeptide out of which the various virus proteins are broken down: this is done by cleavage—a process which is almost certainly carried out by a proteolytic enzyme and which takes place in several stages.

Site of replication: poliovirus replicates and is assembled in the cytoplasm.

REPLICATION OF RNA VIRUSES IN WHICH THE MESSENGER RNA IS COMPLEMENTARY TO THE INPUT RNA

Most of the large enveloped RNA viruses belong to this category: the group includes influenza, parainfluenza and mumps viruses.

Transcriptase: viruses of this group contain a RNA-dependent RNA polymerase within the infecting particles: this enzyme transcribes messenger RNA off the input strand

of virus RNA: with parainfluenza and mumps viruses this is a single strand of RNA but influenza virus has a fragmented genome which consists of 7 separate pieces of RNA.
Virus structural proteins: some of the structural proteins are glycoproteins which form part of the virus envelope: in the case of influenza virus the structural proteins include the protein part of the ribonucleoprotein core of the virus in addition to the haemagglutinin and neuraminidase which are part of the virus envelope.
Site of replication: influenza proteins are synthesised in the cytoplasm and some are transported into the nucleus for assembly into nucleocapsids: the nucleocapsids then move back into the cytoplasm and acquire an envelope by budding through the cell plasma membrane: during infection the membrane becomes altered by the appearance within it of the virus haemagglutinin and neuraminidase: these two structural proteins therefore become incorporated into the particles as they are enveloped during release from the cells: the assembly of mumps and parainfluenza viruses follows a similar course except that there does not appear to be a nuclear phase.

Further Reading

Baltimore, D. (1971). Expression of animal virus genomes. *Bact. Rev.* **35,** 235.

Strategy of the Viral Genome. *A Ciba Foundation Symposium.* Edited by G. E. W. Wolstenholme and Maeve O'Connor. Churchill Livingstone. Edinburgh 1971.

CHAPTER III

LABORATORY DIAGNOSIS OF VIRUS INFECTIONS

WITH a few exceptions, the diagnosis of most viral infections in the laboratory is slow and the patient is often convalescent before a result is available.

Laboratory diagnosis is therefore of limited use in the case of the individual patient—but it is of great importance in medical and especially epidemiological research: an exception to this is smallpox in which laboratory diagnosis is rapid and is an important factor in helping to control outbreaks of infection.

Laboratory virological diagnosis depends on three principal techniques:—

Isolation of virus

Serology—demonstration of antibody to virus

Direct demonstrations of virus or virus antigen in smears from lesions.

ISOLATION

Isolation is a widely used method of diagnosing infection and is usually quicker than serology.

However *viruses are sometimes carried by healthy people* so that isolation *per se* does not necessarily mean that the virus isolated has caused the disease under investigation.

Specimens:

Body secretions or excretions or other material from lesions or sites where virus is commonly present:

If collected on a swab, a wooden-shafted swab should be used and the tip broken off into a small bottle of transport medium—usually tissue culture medium—to preserve the virus.

Specimens should be delivered to the laboratory as quickly as possible after collection: If possible specimens should be kept cold, *i.e.* at 4° C. during delivery.

If specimens are contaminated with bacteria (*e.g.* faeces and throat swabs) antibiotics are added in the laboratory. They are then centrifuged at low speeds to deposit the bacteria (the slowly sedimenting virus particles remaining in the supernate).

Three main systems are inoculated for virus isolation:—

1. Tissue culture
2. Chick embryo
3. Laboratory animals.

Tissue Culture

Cells from man or animals are grown in a single layer (or monolayer) on the walls of test tubes or on one side of flat bottles. Cultures of cells are usually incubated at 36·5°C.

Tissue culture growth medium is basically a balanced salt solution containing the following substances:—

Glucose—main energy source

Serum—usually calf, sometimes human or horse

Protein supplement—lactalbumen hydrolysate

Penicillin and streptomycin to prevent bacterial contamination

Sodium bicarbonate as buffer: the pH should be between 7·2 and 7·4.

Media are sometimes enriched with solutions of amino acids and vitamins.

Three main types of tissue cultures are used in virology:—

1. **Primary cultures:**

   Prepared by dispersing cells with trypsin from tissue fragments: there is little cell division during growth in culture—cells merely settle and spread out on the glass to form a monolayer or single layer of cells. After two to three weeks the cells degenerate and are discarded.

   e.g. monkey kidney and human amnion cells.

2. **Semi-continuous cell strains:**

   The cells are usually fibroblasts derived from embryo tissues: they have a diploid number of chromosomes.

   There is a rapid growth rate and the cells can be subcultured up to about 50 passages in culture.

   e.g. human embryo lung strains.

3. **Continuous cell lines:**

   Usually derived from malignant or cancerous tissue: the cells are often—although not always—epithelial: the chromosomes are heteroploid. There is a rapid growth rate and the cells can be subcultured indefinitely.

   e.g. HeLa cells (derived from a cervical cancer).

Virus growth is recognised by development of:—

1. *CPE*

   (cytopathic effect): cell degeneration or death: usually recognised by rounding of the cells—sometimes with shrinkage but with other viruses the cells are large and show ' ballooning ': as the cells die many detach from the glass. Some viruses produce syncytia or multinucleated giant cells.

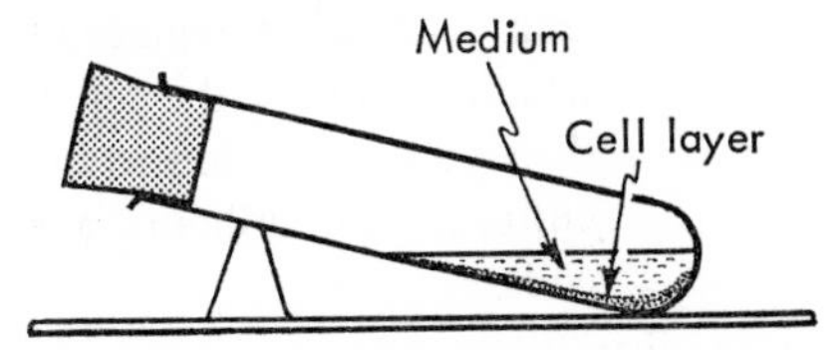

Test tube containing tissue culture: incubated in slightly tilted position so that cells settle and grow up one side of tube.

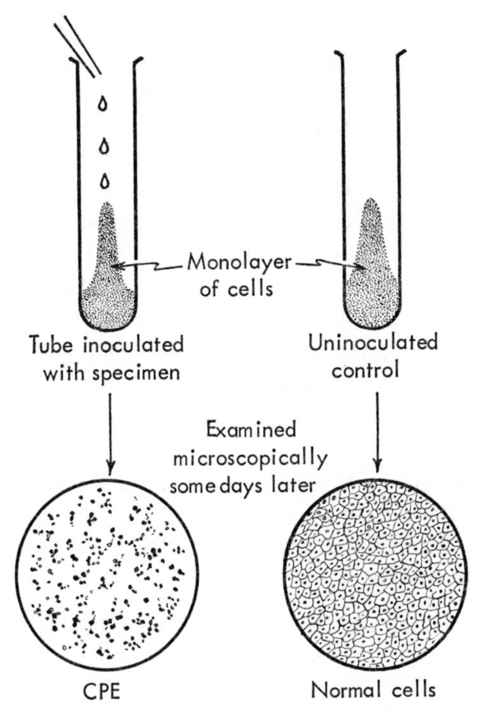

FIG. 1
Diagram showing inoculation of tissue culture for viral isolation.

2. *Haemadsorption*: seen with haemagglutinating viruses which mature at the cell surface. Erythrocytes are added to infected tissue cultures and adhere to the infected cells.
3. *Fluorescence*: virus antigen is detected in infected cells by fluorescence due to an antigen-antibody reaction between virus and antiviral serum. In the *direct technique,* the antiviral serum is labelled with a fluorescent dye: in the more widely used *indirect technique,* application of unlabelled antiviral serum is followed by labelled antibody to gamma globulin: in the indirect technique, the virus fluoresces due to a reaction between the labelled antiserum and the viral antibody which in turn has reacted and become attached to the virus antigen in the infected cells.
4. *Interference*: the cells appear normal but are no longer susceptible to superinfection with CPE-producing viruses.

The virus is typed by testing for inhibition of these effects in tissue culture with standard antiviral sera except in the case of fluorescence which is itself an immunologically-specific technique.

Cytopathic viruses: The most widely used test is for *neutralisation of infectivity.*

Neutralisation tests can be used with any virus which produces CPE in tissue cultures: known or standard antiviral serum is tested with the unknown virus: if the antiserum reacts specifically with the virus, it neutralises infectivity—and therefore prevents the usual CPE produced by the virus: the virus is thus identified since it has been shown to be identical to the virus against which the standard antiviral serum was prepared.

The neutralising antigen of the virus is contained in the protein coat of the virus particle.

Neutralisation Test

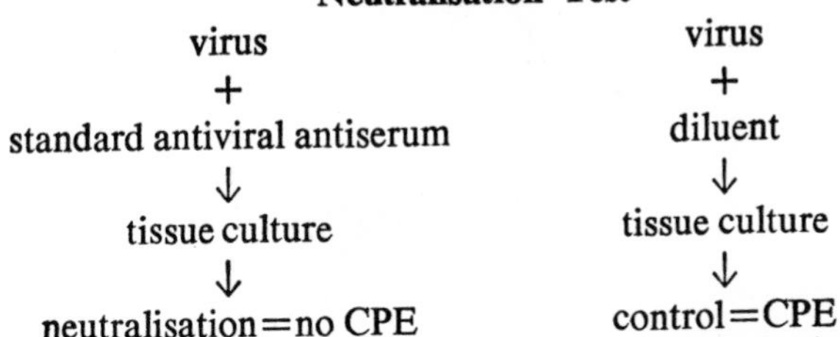

Haemadsorbing viruses are typed or identified by testing for neutralisation by standard antiserum of the ability of the virus to haemadsorb or for haemagglutination-inhibition using the virus released into the medium as the source of haemagglutinin.

Interference-producing viruses are typed by testing for serological inhibition of the interference.

Chick Embryo

Fertile hens' eggs were widely used before the advent of the tissue culture technique but have now been largely replaced by tissue cultures for virus isolation. Chick embryos are susceptible to far fewer viruses than tissue cultures.

There are three main routes of inoculation:—

1. Onto the chorio-allantoic membrane
2. Into the amniotic cavity
3. Into the allantoic cavity.

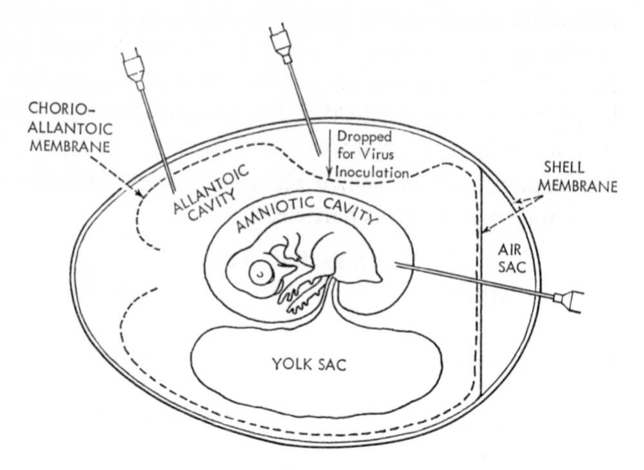

FIG. 2
Diagram of chick embryo showing routes of inoculation for viral isolation.

Embryos are used aged from 7-12 days: the optimal age for each route of inoculation depends on the development of the tissues *e.g.* the amnion is maximal at 10-12 days.

Virus growth is recognised by the development of:—

1. *Pocks* on the chorio-allantoic membrane.
2. *Haemagglutinin* in the amniotic or allantoic cavities: erythrocytes are added to serial dilutions of the fluid and observed for haemagglutination (Fig. 3).

   Agglutinated erythrocytes spread out to cover the bottom of the container.

   Non-agglutinated erythrocytes pack into a small button in the bottom of the container.

The virus is typed by testing the isolate with standard antisera for:—

1. Reduction in number of pocks produced

2. Inhibition of viral haemagglutination
3. Complement fixation.

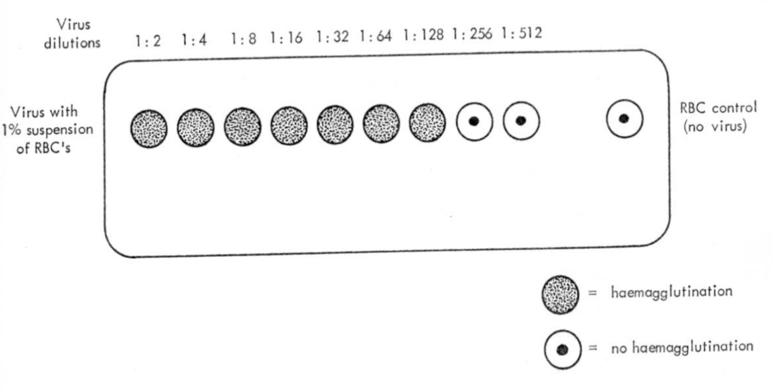

FIG. 3
Diagram of haemagglutination test for virus. Titre of virus haemagglutinin is 128.

LABORATORY ANIMALS

Animals are required for the isolation of some viruses. After inoculation animals are observed for signs of disease or death.

Viruses which can only be isolated in laboratory animals are identified by testing for neutralisation by standard antiserum of the viral pathogenicity for the animals or by haemagglutination-inhibition in the case of haemagglutinating viruses.

SEROLOGY

Infection is diagnosed by the demonstration of the development of virus antibody at the same time as the patient's illness.

Specimens: two samples of blood
—the first taken in the acute phase of illness
—the second taken 10-14 days later in convalescence.

The acute and convalescent serum samples are tested in parallel to detect a *rise in titre* of antibodies to the virus.

Titre is the highest dilution of antiserum at which activity is demonstrated: it is usually expressed as the reciprocal of the serum dilution *e.g.* 64 instead of 1/64.

Tests are regarded as indicating recent infection by:—

1. *4-fold or greater rise in antibody titre* from the acute to the convalescent serum samples.
2. *A stationary but high titre* of antibodies in both samples.
3. *A fall in titre* of antibodies can sometimes be regarded as evidence of recent infection.

Three main serological tests are used to detect antibodies:—

Complement fixation tests.
Haemagglutination-inhibition tests.
Neutralisation tests.

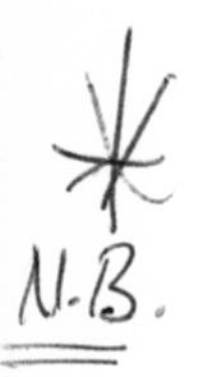

1. **Complement Fixation Tests**

Very widely used and the most useful of the serological tests available. Based on the fact that when an antigen-antibody reaction takes place complement (a complex constituent of animal sera) is 'fixed' or used up. Complement is heat-labile.

Most viruses are good complement-fixing antigens.

The test is carried out in two stages.

Test:—

Stage 1 Dilutions of patient's serum are mixed with virus and complement (guinea-pig serum is used as a source of complement) and left at 4°C. overnight.

Stage 2 An indicator system is added to demonstrate the presence or absence (*i.e.* fixation) of complement.

The indicator system used is of sheep erythrocytes sensitised by mixing with haemolysin (antibody to sheep erythrocytes): in the presence of complement the haemolysin lyses the erythrocytes but cannot do so if complement has been fixed or used up in Stage 1.

Result. The test (Fig. 4) is read as follows:—

HAEMOLYSIS of indicator system	NO HAEMOLYSIS of indicator system
↓	↓
means that complement is present (*i.e.* has not been used up in Stage 1)	means that complement has been used up in Stage 1
↓	↓
Therefore:— no antigen-antibody reaction has taken place at Stage 1.	*Therefore*:— an antigen-antibody reaction has taken place at Stage 1.
Conclusion: no antibody is present in the patient's serum.	*Conclusion*: antibody is present in the patient's serum.

2. **Haemagglutination-inhibition tests**

Not so widely used for demonstration of antibody because:—

1. Non-specific inhibitors of haemagglutination are common in patients' sera and may obscure genuine specific inhibition.

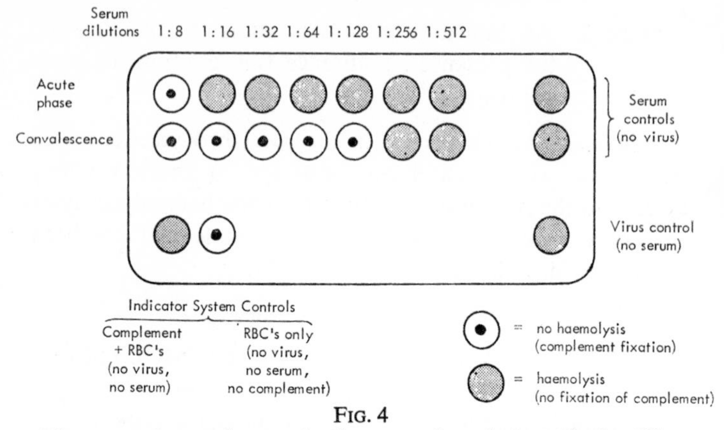

FIG. 4

Diagram of complement-fixation test for viral antibody. Virus antigen is mixed overnight at 4°C. with dilutions of the patient's serum and complement before addition of sensitised sheep erythrocytes. Titre of complement-fixing antibody has risen from 8 in the acute phase to 128 in convalescence—a greater than 4-fold rise in titre indicating recent infection.

2. The reaction is often very strain-specific (so that antibody reacts in high titre only with the homologous strain of virus).

Non-specific inhibitors—if present—must be removed before testing by treatment with trypsin or periodate.

In the test, dilutions of the patient's serum are mixed with a standard dose of the haemagglutinating virus and left to react for one hour: suitable erythrocytes are then added. After an hour or two at a suitable temperature, the test is read by observing the settling patterns of the erythrocytes (Fig. 5).

3. **Neutralisation Tests**

More time-consuming and extravagant of materials than the other two tests.

Dilutions of the serum are tested for neutralisation of a standard virus preparation.

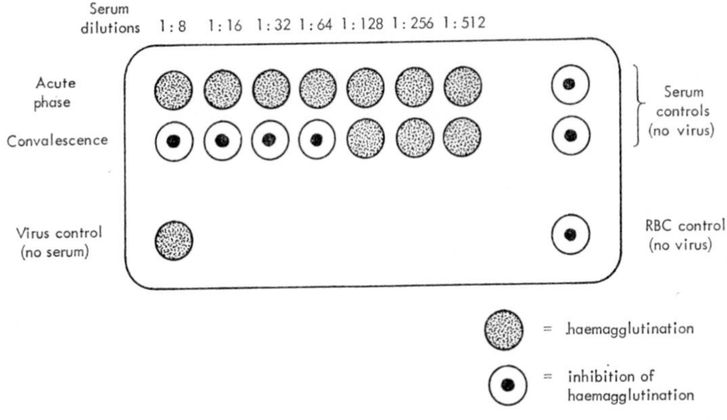

FIG. 5

Diagram of haemagglutination-inhibition test for viral antibody. The haemagglutinating virus is mixed with dilutions of the patient's serum for 1 hour before addition of erythrocytes. Titre of haemagglutination-inhibiting antibody has risen from less than 8 in the acute phase to 64 in convalescence—a greater than 4-fold rise in titre indicating recent infection.

DIRECT DEMONSTRATION OF VIRUS

The electron microscope is now being increasingly used to demonstrate virus particles in skin lesions: this shows the structure of the particle in sufficient detail to distinguish, for example, pox group viruses from herpes group viruses: it is only successful where large numbers of particles (*e.g.* 10^9 particles per ml.) are present: failure to demonstrate particles does not exclude the diagnosis of viral infection.

Fluorescent-antibody tests: detection of virus in smears of lesions by demonstrating specific fluorescence with standard antiviral serum (see p. 20). This technique—like electron microscopy—gives a rapid diagnosis but does not require such high titres of virus in the specimen. Non-specific staining may be a problem and careful contrc are essential to avoid false positive results.

Immunodiffusion: virus antigen may also be detected by precipitation reaction against antiviral serum in agar ge this is a relatively rapid means of detecting virus in a spe men and takes from 2 to 6 hours.

INCLUSION BODIES

Inclusion bodies are acidophilic or basophilic-staini masses seen in the nucleus or cytoplasm of infected cel Some are composed of virus particles which may be pa tially masked by ground substance: others are hom geneous and may be a non-specific sequel to cell dama rather than due to the presence of virus particles.

FURTHER READING

GRIST, N. R., ROSS, C. A. C., BELL, E. J. & STOTT, E. J. (196 *Diagnostic Methods in Clinical Virology*. Oxford: Blackwell.

CHAPTER IV

INFLUENZA

INFLUENZA is one of the great epidemic diseases. From time to time, influenza becomes pandemic and sweeps literally throughout the world. The most severe pandemic recorded was in the winter of 1918 to 1919, when more than 10 million people perished. World-wide pandemics of influenza are due to the emergence of antigenically new strains of influenza virus to which there is no pre-existing immunity.

CLINICAL FEATURES

Influenza is an acute febrile illness which is associated with considerable malaise and variable but often minor respiratory symptoms (such as cough). In uncomplicated cases the illness lasts for 3-4 days: some—perhaps many—cases of influenzal infection are *symptomless*. Influenza is usually *limited to the epithelium of the respiratory tract* and the infection does not become generalised throughout the body: attacks are often followed by lassitude and depression.

Complications

In a small proportion of cases, the acute infection progresses to a severe *influenzal pneumonia*: this has a high mortality rate and is the usual cause of death in influenza. It is often—but not always—associated with a secondary infection of the lungs by bacteria such as *Staphylococcus aureus* or *Haemophilus influenzae*.

Route of infection

Inhalation of respiratory secretions from an infected person.

Primary site of virus multiplication is the superficial epithelium of the upper and lower respiratory tract: influenza causes damage to the cilia and desquamation of the epithelium.

Epidemiology

Seasonal distribution

The highest incidence of infection is during the winter (but the epidemic of ' Asian ' influenza started in Britain in the summer of 1957).

Spread

This is more rapid than in any other infectious disease: in addition to other important properties, influenza virus possesses an inherent and marked capacity for rapid spread.

Pandemic infection

This breaks out every 30-40 years: thus pandemics were recorded in 1847, 1889-90, 1918-19 and in 1957.

Antigenic variation

The capacity of influenza virus for rapid spread is greatly enhanced by its tendency to undergo antigenic variation.

Major antigenic variation also takes place from time to time and when this happens the new virus is unaffected by existing antibody to the old virus strain: since there is no immunity to the new virus among the population at large, it is able to spread and infect on a wide scale: the first influenza A virus, A/PR/8/34, was isolated in 1934 and remained the predominant infecting strain until the emergence of the strain A/FM/1/47 in 1947: this strain predominated until 1957 when 'Asian' influenza due to strain A/Singapore/1/57 appeared: in 1968, a variant, A/Hong Kong/1/68 emerged also from the Far East but antigenically different enough from A/Singapore/1/57 to spread fairly widely in the community: the 'Hong Kong' variant has caused three widespread epidemics in Britain—the first and mild one in the early months of 1969, the second and more severe in the winter of 1969-70 and the third in the winter of 1971-72.

Minor antigenic variation or *antigenic drift* is commonly seen from season to season but the existing antibody levels in the population usually provide sufficient immunity to prevent a large outbreak.

VIROLOGY

1. Myxoviruses ('myxo'=affinity for mucin)
2. RNA viruses
3. Roughly spherical particles with an envelope which is derived from the host cell and contains radially-projecting spikes of virus haemagglutinin and neuraminidase; inside the envelope is helically coiled ribonucleoprotein (Fig. 6)
4. Medium size, 80-100 nm
5. Sensitive to ether
6. Haemagglutinate erythrocytes of various animal species
7. Grow in amniotic cavity of the chick embryo and—after passage or subculture—in the allantoic cavity also

8. Grow in monkey kidney tissue culture with haema sorption.

There are three influenza viruses A, B and C which ca be differentiated by complement fixation test:—

A—the principal cause of epidemic influenza

B—usually associated with a milder disease but can als cause winter epidemics

C—low or doubtful pathogenicity for man.

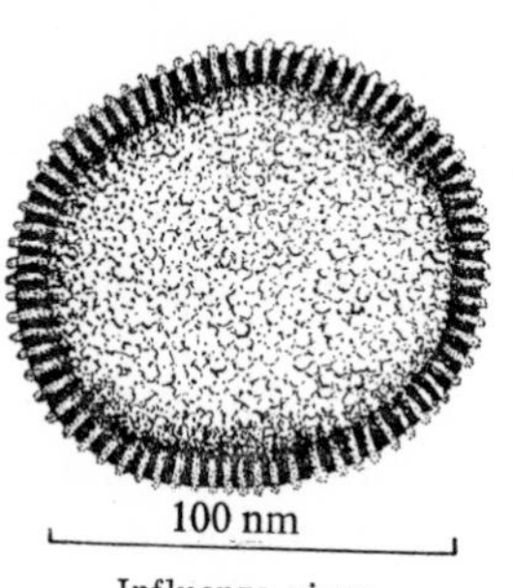

Influenza virus

FIG. 6

Antigenic structure

Influenza viruses have three main antigens:—

1. *"S" or soluble antigen*—the ribonucleoprotein core c the virus particle: this antigen is type specific in tha all influenza A viruses share a common S antigen whic is different to that shared by all influenza B viruses demonstrated by complement fixation test.
2. *Haemagglutinin*: contained in the radially-projectin spikes in the virus envelope: strain-specific: the mai neutralising antigen responsible for immunity of th virus.
3. *Neuraminidase*: an enzyme also contained in the viru envelope: plays a minor role in immunity to reinfection

Antigenic variation

Major antigenic change is due to the emergence of a new strain of virus containing either a new haemagglutinin or neuraminidase or both: this is illustrated by the serological types of haemagglutinin and neuraminidase contained in the major influenza virus A strains:—

	Haemagglutinin	*Neuraminidase*
A/PR/8/34	H0	N1
A/FM/1/47	H1	N1
A/Singapore/1/57	H2	N2
A/Hong Kong/1/68	H3	N2

Genetic recombination: because of its fragmented genome, influenza virus shows a high rate of recombination during replication: there is evidence that new human strains of influenza virus A can arise by recombination with avian and animal strains of influenza virus A: as a result, a new virus emerges which has acquired by recombination, genetic material which codes for a new haemagglutinin or neuraminidase and which has been derived from an animal virus strain.

Haemagglutination by Influenza Viruses

Haemagglutination is due to adsorption of influenza virus particles to specific receptors on the erythrocyte surface.

Receptors are composed of muco-polysaccharide—neuraminic acid.

Virus haemagglutinin is contained on the radially-projecting spikes in the envelope round the virus particle: the haemagglutinin is a combining site which is antigenic and which has an affinity for neuraminic acid:

Neuraminidase: influenza virus particles also contain an enzyme which is similar in action to the receptor destroying enzyme (RDE) of *Vibrio cholerae*: this destroys the neuraminic acid receptors on erythrocytes: after viral haemagglutination, if the mixture of virus and erythrocytes is kept at 37° C., the neuraminidase causes the virus to elute from the erythrocytes; as a result the haemagglutination is reversed and the erythrocytes disperse again.

Haemagglutination-inhibition. Treatment of the virus with specific antibody prevents haemagglutination: haemagglutination-inhibition is *strain-specific i.e.* haemagglutination by a new virus strain, *e.g.* the A/Singapore/1/57 strain of 'Asian' influenza, is unaffected by antibody to older strains of virus A.

(In contrast, all A strains cross-react in complement fixation tests due to their sharing the common group A complement-fixing antigen.)

Phase variation. In the laboratory, after passage of culture, influenza viruses sometimes undergo variation in their reaction in haemagglutination-inhibition tests (using antisera to different strains within the same group of influenza viruses).

P phase virus—strongly inhibited by homologous antiserum only

Q phase virus—poorly inhibited by any antisera (including homologous)

R phase virus—strongly inhibited by heterologous and homologous antisera.

Diagnosis

Isolation

Specimens: mouth washings and throat swabs

Inoculate. 1. *Monkey kidney tissue cultures*

Observe: for haemadsorption of human group O erythrocytes

Virus is typed: by testing for inhibition of haemadsorption by specific antisera

2. *Amniotic cavity of chick embryo*

Observe for haemagglutination of fowl erythrocytes: the titre of haemagglutination for fowl erythrocytes is often initially low but increases on passage in the allantoic cavity: this is known as O (original) → D (derived) variation

Virus is typed by testing for inhibition of haemagglutination with standard antisera.

Serology

COMPLEMENT FIXATION TEST: with the *'S' or soluble antigen*—the ribonucleoprotein from the centre of the virus particle: this antigen is *type-specific i.e.* all strains of virus A have the same 'S' antigen.

Complement fixation tests to demonstrate antibody to influenza virus are carried out by testing sera against the 'S' antigens of viruses A and B

HAEMAGGLUTINATION-INHIBITION TESTS

Antibody to influenza viruses can also be demonstrated by testing patients' sera for inhibition of haemagglutination: since the reaction is strain-specific, tests must be made with currently circulating strains of virus.

VACCINES

Because of the considerable morbidity and the risk of fatal complications, vaccines have been developed against influenza viruses.

At the time of a pandemic, the speed with which new strains of influenza virus spread makes it difficult if not impossible to prepare sufficient quantities of vaccine in time to protect any but a few key workers.

There are two types of influenza vaccine:—

Inactivated virus vaccines: administered by subcutaneous injection: saline suspension of virus grown in the allantoic cavity of the chick embryo; a relatively large amount of virus is required to give an adequate antibody response.

In general, influenza vaccines give relatively short-lived immunity—usually lasting only a few months. At best the protection conferred is of the order of 60 per cent.

A similar vaccine combined with mineral oil adjuvant has also been investigated. The antibody-response is stronger and longer-lasting and less virus is therefore required for vaccine production: sterile abscesses at the site of injection are sometimes seen and the vaccine is not in general use.

Purified haemagglutinin: vaccines containing haemagglutinin from disrupted virus particles are also under trial:

Live attenuated virus vaccine: administered intra-nasally. There have been some promising results but difficulties in achieving standardisation and stabilisation have still to be overcome.

Further Reading

Stuart-Harris, C. H. (1965). *Influenza and Other Virus Infections of the Respiratory Tract*, 2nd ed. London: Arnold.

CHAPTER V

UPPER RESPIRATORY TRACT INFECTIONS

VIRUS infections of the respiratory tract are extremely common: they are a major cause of sickness and absence from work and therefore of great economic importance.

The main groups of viruses which affect the upper respiratory tract are shown in Table III.

TABLE III

VIRUSES WHICH AFFECT THE UPPER RESPIRATORY TRACT

VIRUS GROUP	NO. OF SEROTYPES	DISEASE
Adenoviruses	33	pharyngitis and conjunctivitis
Parainfluenza viruses	4	croup: colds, lower respiratory infections in children
Respiratory syncytial virus	1	bronchiolitis and pneumonia in infants, colds in older children
Rhinoviruses	89	colds
Coronaviruses	?	colds
Coxsackieviruses	2 (types A21, B3)	colds
Echoviruses	2 (types 11, 20)	colds

ADENOVIRUSES

Clinical Features

Clinically, the main symptoms of adenovirus respiratory infection are:—

pharyngitis and conjunctivitis

but the syndromes associated with adenoviruses are ill-defined (Table IV).

Table IV

SYNDROMES ASSOCIATED WITH ADENOVIRUSES

Syndrome	Adenovirus types
1. *Epidemic infection* pharyngo-conjunctival fever febrile catarrh acute respiratory disease	3, 4, 7, 14
2. *Endemic infection* pharyngitis follicular conjunctivitis	1, 2, 3, 5, 6, 7
3. *Epidemic kerato-conjunctivitis* 'shipyard eye'	8

1. *Epidemic infection*: common in recruit camps where attack rates of 70 per cent. have been reported; also seen in children's institutions: due to crowding together of susceptible young hosts.
2. *Endemic infection*: adenovirus infections are endemic in the general population; however they usually constitute less than 5 per cent. of the respiratory infections seen in the community at large.
3. *Epidemic kerato-conjunctivitis*: a form of eye infection which is spread mainly by contaminated instruments at eye clinics and surgeries; epidemics are seen in shipyard workers who are prone to minor eye injuries which

require treatment at eye clinics: unlike the other forms of adenovirus disease, this disease is usually associated with only one adenovirus—type 8.

Alimentary tract: adenoviruses are common in the alimentary as well as the respiratory tract; this is probably due to the predilection of adenoviruses for lymphoid tissue: adenoviruses may play a role in:—

1. *mesenteric adenitis*: enlargement of the intestinal lymph glands; a common cause of acute abdominal pain in children.
2. *intussusception*: invagination and telescoping of the gut causing intestinal obstruction in young children: probably due to action of peristalsis on enlarged intestinal lymph glands.

Oncogenic properties: several adenoviruses cause cancer on injection into hamsters: the most highly oncogenic are types 12, 18 and 31: there is no indication so far of any association of adenoviruses with tumours in man.

Latent infection: adenoviruses have a marked tendency to cause latent infection in tissues such as the tonsils and adenoids.

Virology

1. 33 serological types which react independently in neutralisation tests: but all adenoviruses share a common group complement-fixing antigen
2. DNA viruses
3. Medium size: 60-70 nm; icosahedron-shaped particles with spikes topped with knobs projecting from the vertices (Fig. 7)
4. Resistant to ether
5. Most haemagglutinate

6. Grow slowly in tissue cultures *e.g.* HeLa cells or human embryonic cells, with CPE of clusters of rounded and ' ballooned ' cells.

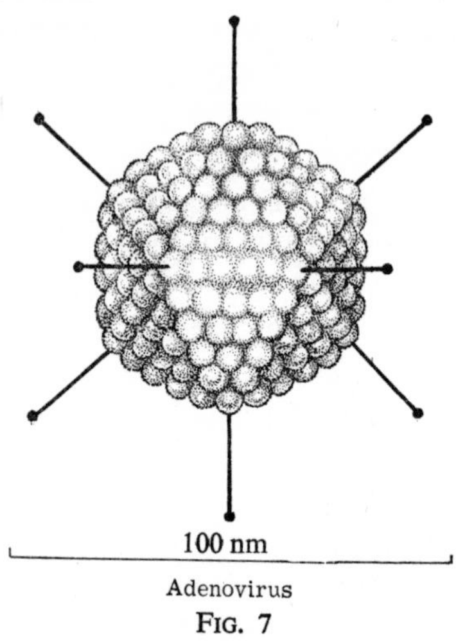

Adenovirus
FIG. 7

DIAGNOSIS

Isolation

Specimens: mouth washings, throat swabs, faeces

Inoculate: human embryonic cell cultures or HeLa cells

Observe: for characteristic CPE of large rounded cells arranged like ' bunches of grapes '.

Type virus in stages:—

1. Confirm as an adenovirus by *complement fixation test* with standard antiserum
2. Adenoviruses can be subdivided into groups by testing for *haemagglutination* with rat and rhesus monkey erythrocytes:

Main adenovirus types	*erythrocytes*	
	rat	*rhesus*
3, 7, 14	0	+
8	+	+
1, 2, 4, 5, 6	±	0

± = partial haemagglutination

3. Having grouped the adenovirus, it is typed by *neutralisation* with appropriate standard antisera.

Serology

COMPLEMENT FIXATION TEST: All adenoviruses share a common group complement-fixing antigen (although they have different antigens in neutralisation tests).

By testing patients' sera against adenovirus group antigen in complement fixation tests, adenovirus infection can be diagnosed: but this gives no indication of the serotype of the adenovirus responsible.

PARAINFLUENZA VIRUSES

CLINICAL FEATURES

Parainfluenza viruses cause *respiratory disease that is between influenza and the common cold in severity*: they are the main cause of *croup* (acute laryngo-tracheo-bronchitis): the highest attack rates are in children under 5 years old; infection is also common in school children but is less common in adults.

VIROLOGY

1. Paramyxoviruses: 4 serological types
2. RNA viruses
3. Rather large, about 100-200 nm
4. Haemagglutinate human group O erythrocytes
5. Grow in monkey kidney tissue cultures with haemadsorption.

Diagnosis

Isolation

Specimens: mouth washings, throat swabs

Inoculate: monkey kidney tissue cultures

Observe: for haemadsorption with human group O erythrocytes (CPE is variable and slow)

Type virus: by testing for inhibition of haemadsorption by standard antisera.

Serology

Complement fixation test: not very useful: frequent cross-reactions with other paramyxoviruses may make interpretation difficult.

RESPIRATORY SYNCYTIAL VIRUS

Clinical Features

Main cause in infants of *bronchiolitis* (a severe form of bronchitis with respiratory distress) and *pneumonia*—both of which may be fatal: it also causes common colds in children over 2 years old.

Mainly attacks children under 5 years old; peak incidence is in infants under 1 year old; rare in adults.

Virology

1. RNA virus
2. One serological type
3. Medium size, 90-130 nm
4. Grows in HeLa cells with syncytial CPE
5. Does not haemagglutinate

Diagnosis

Isolation

Specimens: Mouth washings, nasal secretions (*not* frozen during delivery because the virus is inactivated by freezing)

Inoculate: the ' Bristol ' line of HeLa cells

Observe: for characteristic CPE of syncytia of multinucleated giant-cells

Type virus: by complement fixation test with standard antiserum.

Serology

Complement fixation test.

RHINOVIRUSES

Clinical Features

Rhinoviruses are the main cause of *common colds*: there are a large number of serologically distinct viruses and therefore no cross immunity so that repeated infections are common.

Rhinovirus infections are more common in children than in adults but adult common colds are more often due to rhinoviruses than to other respiratory viruses.

Rhinoviruses vary slightly in the symptoms they produce, but ' breed true ' in that the same virus tends to produce the same symptoms in different patients.

Common colds have a worldwide distribution and are seen in the tropics as well as in Britain: exposure to low temperatures does not predispose to common colds.

Virology

1. Picornaviruses (pico = small + RNA): 89 recognised serotypes

2. RNA viruses
3. Small, 15-20 nm
4. Resistant to ether
5. Inactivated at acid pH (unlike enteroviruses—the other members of the picornavirus group)
6. Grow in tissue cultures but at 33°C. instead of the usual 37°C. (the temperature of the nostrils is 33°C.)
7. Two groups of viruses:—
   1. 'M' rhinoviruses—grow in monkey kidney tissue culture with CPE
   2. 'H' rhinoviruses—grow only in human embryo cells —with CPE—a larger group than the 'M' viruses.

Diagnosis

Isolation

Specimens: nasal secretions, mouth washings

Inoculate: monkey kidney and human embryo tissue cultures

Observe: for CPE

Type virus: by neutralisation with standard antisera.

Serology

Impractical because of the large number of serological types of rhinovirus.

Note: Laboratory diagnosis of common colds is too time-consuming for routine purposes and is therefore restricted to epidemiological research.

OTHER VIRUSES CAUSING COMMON COLDS:—

Coronaviruses: medium-sized (80-160 nm) RNA viruses which are ether-sensitive: the virus particles are unusual and resemble those of avian bronchitis and mouse hepatitis: the roughly spherical particles are surrounded by a fringe of rounded or club-shaped projections: isolated in organ cultures of human embryo trachea where virus may be detected by ciliary immobilisation or by electron microscopy of the culture: some strains can be adapted to growth in a line of human embryo lung cells—L132—with CPE.

Enteroviruses: some enteroviruses (see p. 49) may cause respiratory infections: the main viruses associated with respiratory disease are Coxsackievirus A21 (Coe virus), B3 and echoviruses types 11 and 20.

Further Reading

British Medical Journal (1965). Report: M.R.C. working party on acute respiratory virus infections. **2**, 319.

Potter, C. W. (1967). In *Modern Trends in Medical Virology,* ed. Heath, R. B. & Waterson, A. P., **1**, pp. 162-181. London: Butterworths.

Tyrrell, D. A. J. (1965). *Common Colds and Related Diseases.* London: Arnold.

CHAPTER VI

NEUROLOGICAL DISEASE DUE TO VIRUSES

NEUROLOGICAL disease is *a serious and not uncommon complication of virus infection.* Most human pathogenic viruses are capable of spreading to the central nervous system (CNS). Virus lesions in the CNS are due mainly to *viral multiplication* in the cells of the nervous tissues with cellular damage and dysfunction and consequent neurological signs and symptoms. But the *immune response of the host* may also play a role in causing lesions. Lesions may be due to an antigen-antibody reaction in the tissues—with resulting inflammatory response—rather than to virus multiplication alone. In one form of viral CNS disease (post-infectious encephalomyelitis) virus cannot be isolated from the CNS.

Most viruses *invade* the CNS by *the blood stream* but some, *e.g.* rabies, reach the CNS by the *neural route* as a result of spreading along the peripheral nerves.

CNS involvement is not always followed by neurological disease—there is evidence that *symptomless involvement of the CNS* is common in measles and mumps.

Viral neurological disease falls into four main syndromes:—

1. *encephalitis*: the main symptoms are drowsiness, mental confusion, convulsions, focal neurological signs and sometimes coma.

TABLE V

	Direct invasion of CNS by virus			Virus not demonstrable in CNS: Disease is probably due to abnormal immune response of host to infection
Disease	Encephalitis	Paralysis (anterior poliomyelitis)	Aseptic meningitis	Post-infectious encephalomyelitis
Site	Brain	Anterior horn cells of spinal cord	Meninges	Brain
Lesions	destructive lesions in grey matter; neuronal damage	destructive lesions of lower motor neurones with meningitis	inflammation of meninges, cells in CSF (usually lymphocytes)	perivascular infiltration, microglial proliferation, demyelination
Viruses	herpes simplex togaviruses rabies	enteroviruses (especially polioviruses)	enteroviruses mumps lymphocytic choriomeningitis louping ill	measles vaccinia rubella varicella-zoster

2. *paralysis*: with fever, flaccid paralysis—most often of the lower limbs—and signs of meningitis such as headache with stiffness of neck and back.

3. *aseptic meningitis*: a relatively mild disease with fever, headache and stiffness of neck and back.

4. *post-infectious encephalomyelitis*: with symptoms similar to those of encephalitis.

Table V summarises the main features of the 4 different viral neurological syndromes.

Rare virus neurological syndromes

Viruses also cause other rarer forms of neurological disease; these include the chronic progressive diseases:—

i *Subacute sclerosing panencephalitis* (see p. 86)

ii *Progressive multifocal leucoencephalopathy* (see p. 125).

Although the causal agent has not been firmly identified as a virus, *kuru and Jakob-Creutzfeldt disease* (p. 115) are examples of chronic neurological diseases which are probably viral in origin.

CHAPTER VII

ENTEROVIRUS INFECTIONS; REOVIRUSES

	Enteroviruses			
	polioviruses	*Coxsackieviruses**		*echoviruses†*
		group A	*group B*	
number of serotypes	3	24	6	32

Enteroviruses have the following properties:—

Enter the body via ingestion by mouth.

Primary site of multiplication is the lymphoid tissue of the alimentary tract—including the pharynx.

Spread from the gut is in two directions:—

1. *outwards* into the blood (viraemia) and so to other tissues and organs.
2. *inwards* into the lumen of the gut and to excretion in the faeces.

Important because of their capacity for spread to the CNS with subsequent neurological disease.

Clinical Features

The clinical features are shown in Table VI.

* Coxsackie is the village in New York where these viruses were first isolated.

† Enteric, Cytopathic, Human, Orphan (because originally—but wrongly—thought not to be associated with human disease).

NEUROLOGICAL SYNDROMES

Neurological disease is the most important manifestation of enteroviral infection: it is not associated with one particular group or type of enterovirus.

The illness is usually biphasic: the initial symptoms are of a febrile illness due to viraemia; there is an intervening period of well-being for a day or two followed by the

TABLE VI

DISEASES DUE TO ENTEROVIRUSES

	POLIO-VIRUSES	COXSACKIEVIRUSES GROUP A	COXSACKIEVIRUSES GROUP B	ECHO-VIRUSES
Paralysis	+[1]	+	±	±
Aseptic meningitis	+	+[2]	+	+[2]
Febrile illness	+	+[2]	+	+[2]
Herpangina	−	+	−	−
Hand, foot and mouth disease	−	+	−	−
Bornholm disease	−	−	+	−
Myocarditis and pericarditis	−	−	+	−
Respiratory infections	−	−	±	±

± = reported but rare
[1] = the polioviruses—and especially type 1—are the most paralytogenic enteroviruses
[2] = sometimes associated with a rash

onset of neurological symptoms: these are due to spread of the virus through the 'blood-brain barrier' to invade the CNS.

There are two main types of neurological disease due to enteroviruses:—

1. *Paralysis* or poliomyelitis: an acute illness with pain and *flaccid* paralysis affecting mainly the lower legs: sometimes the muscles of respiration become involved requiring tracheostomy with controlled breathing by positive-pressure respirator: more rarely, the disease may take the form of *bulbar paralysis* when the muscles of breathing and swallowing are primarily involved: paralysis is associated with the signs and symptoms of aseptic meningitis.
   Pathology: paralysis is due to viral damage to the cells of the anterior horn of the spinal cord: this causes lower motor neurone lesions resulting in flaccid paralysis: if damage to the nerve cells is severe, the paralysis may be permanent.
   Paralysis is most often due to the three polioviruses and especially type 1 poliovirus: before the introduction of poliovaccine, epidemics of paralysis were common in countries with a high standard of living *e.g.* U.S.A., Denmark and Australia.
2. *Aseptic meningitis*: signs of neurological disease are present but the damage is minor and there is no paralysis: the main signs and symptoms are fever and headache with nuchal rigidity (stiffness of the neck muscles due to meningeal irritation): lymphocytes and protein in the cerebrospinal fluid (CSF) are increased: the prognosis is good and most patients recover completely—although some minor neurological sequelae have been found in cases followed up after discharge from hospital.

Epidemics of aseptic meningitis are common: these are often due to echovirus type 9 or, before widespread use of poliovaccine, to polioviruses; echoviruses types 4, 6 and 30 and Coxsackieviruses A7, A9 and B5 are also sometimes associated with epidemic aseptic meningitis.

NON-NEUROLOGICAL SYNDROMES

Some non-neurological syndromes are associated with a particular group of enteroviruses.

Herpangina: a painful eruption of vesicles in the mouth and throat: recently, it has been reported as part of the syndrome of 'hand, foot and mouth disease' in which there are vesicles also on the hands and feet: due to group A Coxsackieviruses.

Bornholm disease: also known as pleurodynia or epidemic myalgia: a painful inflammation of muscles which usually involves the intercostal muscles: the disease is named after the Danish island where there was an extensive outbreak in 1930: due to group B Coxsackieviruses.

Myocarditis and pericarditis: acute inflammation of the heart muscle and pericardium due to group B Coxsackieviruses most common in adult males: in the 1965 epidemic of Coxsackievirus B5 infections in England and Wales, 6 per cent. of the patients had cardiac signs or symptoms.

GENERAL FEATURES OF ENTEROVIRUS INFECTIONS

Most enterovirus infections are confined to the alimentary tract and are symptomless.

A small proportion of infections give rise to febrile illness —probably due to viraemia—and this is sometimes accompanied by a rash.

A few cases progress to aseptic meningitis but spread of virus to the CNS is a rare complication of enterovirus infection.

More rarely still, an occasional case develops paralysis: the incidence of paralysis following infection with poliovirus type 1 (the most paralytogenic enterovirus) has been estimated to be of the order of 1 in 100.

EPIDEMIOLOGY

Enterovirus infections are common—especially in children and in conditions of poor hygiene.

Infection is spread mainly by the faecal-oral route from virus excretors to contacts: virus in pharyngeal secretions may also be a source of infection.

Seasonal distribution: infections are far more frequent in the summer than in the winter months.

Predominant strains: one or two enterovirus types usually predominate in a season; the types which emerge are determined by the level of immunity in the population concerned: this in turn depends on the previous infections experienced by the community.

Poor sanitation, e.g. in the under-developed countries, increases the chances of childhood infection so that immunity is acquired early in life.

High standard of living, e.g. in countries such as the U.S.A., diminishes the chance of infection and therefore of immunity being acquired in childhood.

Adults are more liable to develop severe paralysis than children: the risk of developing paralysis is increased by pregnancy, tonsillectomy, fatigue, trauma or inoculation with bacterial vaccines.

Epidemics: countries with a high standard of living have a relatively large proportion of non-immune adults and before the advent of poliovaccines suffered from repeated and widespread epidemics of paralytic disease.

VIROLOGY

1. Picornaviruses (pico=small+RNA)
2. RNA viruses
3. Small, 18-25 nm.
4. Resistant to ether
5. Stable at acid pH (in contrast to the rhinoviruses—the other members of the picornavirus group)
6. Show increased thermal stability at 50°C. for 1 hr. in the presence of molar Mg^{++} or Ca^{++}
7. Most grow in tissue cultures with rapid production of CPE
8. Coxsackieviruses (but not polio or echoviruses) are pathogenic for suckling mice.

DIAGNOSIS

Isolation

Specimens: faeces, throat swabs: CSF is useful for some viruses (*e.g.* echovirus type 9) but not for polioviruses

Inoculate: monkey kidney and human amnion tissue cultures

Observe: for CPE

Type virus: by neutralisation tests with standard antisera; usually done using pooled antisera to reduce the number of tests.

If Coxsackievirus infection is suspected:—

Inoculate: suckling mice intra-peritoneally.

Observe: for characteristic signs of disease:—

1. group A Coxsackieviruses: flaccid paralysis due to widespread myositis.
2. group B Coxsackieviruses: spastic paralysis with tremor due to cerebral lesions: fat-pad necrosis also seen.

Note: Coxsackieviruses of group B grow well in tissue culture so that inoculation of suckling mice is not usually necessary for isolation: it may be used to confirm that a virus isolate has the properties of a group B virus.

Coxsackieviruses of group A, on the other hand, do not grow well in tissue culture, and suckling mice provide a useful method of isolating them.

Significance of enterovirus isolation from faeces:

Symptomless infection of the alimentary tract is common.

Therefore, isolation of virus from faeces is not *proof* that the virus is the cause of the patient's symptoms.

Confirmation can be obtained by demonstrating a rising titre of neutralising antibody to the virus isolated.

The large number of enteroviruses makes serological diagnosis by itself impractical because sera would need to be tested against all or most of them.

Vaccination

Two vaccines are available against the most paralytogenic enteroviruses *i.e.* the three polioviruses.

1. *Sabin live attenuated virus vaccine*—now the main vaccine used for poliomyelitis immunisation.

   Contains the three polioviruses as attenuated strains which have lost neurovirulence for monkeys (*i.e.* ability to produce paralysis or lesions in CNS of monkeys): grown in monkey kidney tissue cultures.

Administered in three oral doses.

Protection: good.

Blood antibody response: good.

Gut immunity: good, vaccinated children show creased resistance to alimentary infection.

Safety: good; strains recovered after passage in hun gut show evidence of a slight shift towards the char teristics of 'wild' virus but this does not appear to ha resulted in disease in contacts.

Vaccinated children are infectious to others so tl vaccine strains may circulate to some extent in community.

Widespread use of this vaccine has resulted in a drama decrease both in paralytic poliomyelitis and in the cir lation of wild polioviruses in the community.

2. *Salk killed virus vaccine*—the first poliovaccine to used on a large scale: although still in use in so countries it is now less widely used than Sabin vacci *Contains* the three polioviruses inactivated by formal hyde: grown in monkey kidney tissue cultures (ea vaccines were contaminated by simian virus SV_{40} wh produces tumours on inoculation into hamsters l there have apparently been no ill-effects in the childı vaccinated).

   Administered by three subcutaneous injections.

   Protection: good, 80-90 per cent. reduction in incideı of paralysis.

   Blood antibody response: good, adequate levels of ne ralising antibody produced.

   Gut immunity: poor, little protection conferred agai alimentary infection.

Safety: good, early accidents were due to inadequate inactivation—now corrected.

REOVIRUSES

(Respiratory Enteric Orphan viruses)

A small group of three viruses which react individually in neutralisation tests but which share a common group complement-fixing antigen: one of the viruses was formerly classified as echovirus type 10.

The properties of reoviruses are similar to those of the enteroviruses: reoviruses are RNA viruses but their RNA is double-stranded: they are larger (60-80 nm.) than enteroviruses, and grow—but relatively slowly—in tissue cultures: they haemagglutinate human erythrocytes and are pathogenic for suckling mice causing lesions similar to those caused by group B coxsackieviruses.

Widespread in cattle and other animals: excretion in animal faeces is common.

Role in human disease: doubtful: reoviruses have been isolated from children with respiratory and gastro-intestinal symptoms but are common in the stools of healthy children also.

Further Reading

British Medical Journal (1961). Report: Poliomyelitis-like disease in 1959. A combined Scottish Study. **2**, 597.

British Medical Journal (1967). Report: Coxsackie B5 virus infections during 1965. **4**, 575.

Scottish Medical Journal (1964). Report: Poliomyelitis-like disease in 1960. A combined Scottish Study, **9**, 141.

CHAPTER VIII

TOGAVIRUS INFECTIONS

(formerly ' arbo-' or arthropod-borne viruses)

TOGAVIRUSES are viruses which are spread by arthropod vectors: the natural hosts are vertebrates (usually birds and small mammals) and the virus is transmitted from animals to man via the bite of an infected arthropod. Togaviruses do not usually cause disease in the vectors which often excrete the virus for many months after infection.

There are more than 200 togaviruses but only about 80 cause disease in man. Togaviruses cause *encephalitis, systemic febrile disease* and *haemorrhagic fever.* Possibly the best-known togavirus—at least historically—is that causing *yellow fever.*

The main medically-important togaviruses are classified into groups in Table VII.

CLINICAL FEATURES

1. *Togavirus encephalitis*: endemic in various areas of the world but not seen in Britain with the exception of the rare disease, louping-ill: epidemics have been reported in the U.S.A., Eastern Europe, Japan, Australia and South America.

The main symptoms of encephalitis are fever, progressively severe headache, nausea, vomiting, stiffness of neck, back and legs, convulsions and sometimes deepening coma: there may be neurological signs such as paralysis and tremor.

Table VII

CLASSIFICATION OF TOGAVIRUSES

Virus	Disease	Vector
Group A		
Eastern Equine Encephalitis	encephalitis	mosquito
Western Equine Encephalitis	encephalitis	mosquito
Venezuelan Equine Encephalitis	encephalitis; febrile disease	mosquito
O'nyong-nyong	febrile disease	mosquito
Chikungunya	febrile disease; haemorrhagic fever	mosquito
Group B		
St. Louis Encephalitis	encephalitis	mosquito
Japanese B Encephalitis	encephalitis	mosquito
Murray Valley Encephalitis	encephalitis	mosquito
Russian Spring Summer Fever	encephalitis	tick
Central European Tick-borne Encephalitis	encephalitis	tick
Louping Ill	encephalitis; meningitis	tick
Yellow Fever	haemorrhagic fever	mosquito
Omsk Haemorrhagic Fever	haemorrhagic fever	tick
Kyasanur Forest Fever	haemorrhagic fever	tick
Dengue	febrile disease and haemorrhagic fever	mosquito
West Nile Fever	febrile disease	mosquito
Bunyamwera Group		
Bunyamwera	febrile disease	mosquito
California Group		
California Encephalitis	encephalitis	mosquito
Phlebotomus Fever Group		
Naples and Sicilian Sandfly Fevers	febrile disease	sandfly (phlebotomus)
Ungrouped		
Colorado Tick Fever	febrile disease	tick
Rift Valley Fever	febrile disease	mosquito

2. *Togavirus systemic febrile disease*: the disease is widel distributed throughout the world and is seen in areas c Africa, the Far East and in Eastern Europe: epidemics c infection have been reported from time to time: the mai symptoms are fever, pain—which is often severe—in th bones and joints, rashes and lymphadenopathy: this grou of syndromes includes *dengue* and *sandfly fever.*

3. *Togavirus haemorrhagic fevers*: are also widely distr buted throughout the world *e.g.* South America, the Fa East, Africa and Russia: the best known example is *yello fever*: the main symptoms of haemorrhagic fevers are c sudden onset of fever, pain in back and limbs, headach prostration and gastro-intestinal upset: haemorrhages fro gums, nose, gastro-intestinal tract, uterus and kidneys ma be seen in severe cases.

4. A considerable proportion of togavirus infections in ma are *symptomless.*

YELLOW FEVER

Clinical Features

Yellow fever varies from a severe hepatitis with a hig mortality rate to a mild febrile illness. The severe diseas is a common form of yellow fever.

The main features of the severe disease are a *biphasi illness*:—

The early phase is characterised by fever, headache nausea and vomiting.

The second phase is of high fever with slow pulse rate jaundice, gastric and other haemorrhages: toxic nephrosi is also common.

Pathology, the principal finding at post-mortem examina tion is severe mid-zonal necrosis of the liver.

EPIDEMIOLOGY

Yellow fever is endemic in areas of Central and South America and across the middle of Africa. Although suitable vectors are present, it is not seen in the Far East.

There are two forms of yellow fever:—

1. *Urban yellow fever*—spread from man to man via mosquitoes breeding in towns and cities: the main host of the disease is man and not some animal vertebrate as in the case of other togavirus infections.

   Vector is the mosquito *Aëdes aegypti.*

   Urban mosquitoes can be readily eradicated by anti-mosquito measures: this type of the disease has therefore been largely brought under control.

2. *Sylvan or jungle yellow fever*—the natural hosts of this form of the disease are wild monkeys and the disease is spread by tree-dwelling mosquitoes: man is an incidental host in the usual monkey to mosquito to monkey cycle: the disease principally affects forest workers and dwellers.

   Vectors are various species of jungle mosquitoes.

   Jungle mosquitoes are impossible to control and this form of yellow fever cannot at present be eradicated.

VIROLOGY

The following are the main properties of togaviruses in general:—

1. RNA viruses
2. Spherical and rod-shaped enveloped particles
3. Wide range of sizes, most are between 30 and 60 nm. but the range is from 17-150 nm.
4. Most haemagglutinate erythrocytes from day-old chicks or geese

5. Pathogenic for suckling mice
6. Grow in tissue culture—some with CPE but some without CPE.

In addition, the virus of yellow fever possesses the following characteristics:—

1. One serological type.
2. Pantropic *i.e.* the virus exhibits both neurotropic and viscerotropic properties: in animals neurotropism predominates, in man viscerotropism (*i.e.*, involvement of liver and kidneys) predominates.

DIAGNOSIS

Isolation

Specimens: blood.

Inoculate: suckling mice intra-cerebrally.

Observe: for tremors, ataxia, paralysis, convulsions or death (5-6 days); at post-mortem look for encephalitis and degeneration of the liver.

Serology

COMPLEMENT FIXATION TESTS.

HAEMAGGLUTINATION-INHIBITION TESTS (of limited value).

Yellow fever:

Post-mortem histology: examination of liver biopsies collected after death by a viscerotome (which can be used by non-medical personnel) has provided a useful method of confirming the diagnosis in fatal cases of yellow fever in areas where there are no virological facilities.

VACCINE

YELLOW FEVER

Contains: live attenuated virus of a strain known as 17D which has been attenuated by repeated passage in chick embryos.

Prepared in chick embryos—early vaccines were almost certainly contaminated by avian leukosis viruses (which cause tumours in fowls) but this has apparently caused no untoward effect in the 30 years in which the vaccine has been used.

Administered in one dose by subcutaneous injection.

Protection conferred: good, solid, long-lasting immunity.

Safety: good, singularly free from side-effects: (the high incidence of jaundice following vaccination of American troops in the last war was shown to be due to contamination of the vaccine by serum hepatitis virus present in the human serum used in manufacture of the vaccine).

Further Reading

World Health Organization (1967). Arboviruses and human disease. *Tech. Rep. Ser. Wld Hlth Org.* **No. 369.**

CHAPTER IX

RHABDOVIRUSES; ARENOVIRUSES

RABIES

RABIES is a severe form of encephalitis due to a virus which affects a wide variety of animal species: rabies is transmitted to man via the bite of an infected animal which is usually—but not always—a dog.

CLINICAL FEATURES

The incubation period is long—usually from 4-12 weeks but sometimes much longer: if the wound is on the head or neck the incubation period is shorter than for wounds on the limbs.

Virus spread from the wound to the CNS is via the nerves.

Symptoms: mainly of excitement, with tremor, muscular contractions and convulsions: spasm of the muscles of swallowing is a common feature (hence the older name for the disease of 'hydrophobia' or fear of water): there is often increased sensitivity of the sensory nervous system.

Prognosis: the disease is nearly always fatal: death often follows a convulsion.

Pathology: despite the severity of the clinical disease, lesions in the CNS are minimal with little evidence of destructive effect on cells: the main changes are the typical intra-cytoplasmic inclusions known as Negri bodies.

Another type of rabies is seen in the West Indies, and Central and South America: this takes the form of *ascend-*

ing myelitis with paralysis and lesions are found in the ganglion cells of the spinal cord: it is spread by the bite of infected vampire bats.

Epidemiology

Rabies is a natural infection of dogs, cats, bats and carnivorous wild animals such as foxes, wolves, skunks and the mongoose family: it is sometimes seen in cattle and wild birds.

Virus is present in the saliva of infected animals—sometimes for up to four days before the onset of symptoms of the disease: animals which remain healthy for seven days after biting can be regarded as being free of virus at the time of biting.

Incidence of rabies after biting: only about 30-40 per cent. of people bitten by a rabid animal develop the disease: rabies is more common after bites on the head or neck than after wounds on the limbs.

Britain is at present free from indigenous rabies: rabies used to be present in animals in Britain but was eradicated by 1921: the strict six month-quarantine laws for animals imported into Britain have on the whole been successful in keeping out the disease.

In 1969, there were two cases of rabies in dogs imported into Britain in which the incubation period had been longer than six months: in the case of one dog, the wild life in the area where the dog had lived on release from quarantine had to be slaughtered: this was to prevent the establishment of a reservoir of infection in wild animals: had this happened, it would have been extremely difficult to eradicate the infection.

Rabies is present in wild animals in Europe, U.S.A. and most other areas of the world.

Virology

1. Bullet-shaped enveloped particles containing helically-coiled nucleo-protein: length 180 nm, diameter 70-80 nm
2. One serological type
3. RNA virus
4. Haemagglutinates goose erythrocytes
5. Grows in hamster kidney and chick embryo cell tissue cultures with eosinophilic cytoplasmic inclusions but usually without CPE
6. Pathogenic for mice and other laboratory animals.

Diagnosis

Isolation

Specimens: brain tissue, saliva, CSF, urine

Inoculate: suckling mice intra-cerebrally

Observe: for paralysis, convulsions; Negri bodies in brain. *If rabies is suspected in an animal* it should be kept under observation to see if the disease develops, and not killed right away: if killed before death due to the disease, Negri bodies may not have developed in sufficient numbers to be detected in histological sections.

Direct Examination of Brain

Impression smears of the Ammon's horn of the hippocampus are examined in two ways:—

1. *With Seller's stain* for red intra-cytoplasmic inclusions or Negri bodies.
2. *By immunofluorescence* (using the direct technique) to demonstrate rabies virus antigen.

Vaccination

Rabies vaccine was first developed by Pasteur in 1885; it consisted of virus attenuated by drying the spinal cords of infected rabbits for varying lengths of time over KOH. Wild rabies virus is known as ' street ' virus and attenuated virus as ' fixed ' virus.

The long incubation period makes rabies a suitable disease for prophylactic immunisation after exposure:

After exposure—or suspicion of exposure—to rabies, patients should be given combined passive and active immunisation.

Passive immunisation: injection of anti-rabies serum prepared in horses.

Active immunisation: two main vaccines are in use:—

1. **Semple vaccine**

   contains: virus inactivated by phenol.

   prepared: from virus in infected rabbit brain tissue.

   administered: by a series of 14 daily subcutaneous injections with boosters at 10 days and 20 days after the last daily dose.

   protection: apparently effective.

   safety: allergic encephalomyelitis sometimes follows immunisation and is due to the repeated injections of nervous tissue.

2. **Duck embryo killed virus vaccine**

   contains: inactivated virus.

   prepared: in duck embryos: although a crude tissue emulsion, it contains very little nervous tissue.

   administered: subcutaneously daily for 14 consecutive days with booster doses at 10 days and 20 days after the last daily dose.

   protection: apparently effective although slightly less potent than brain tissue vaccine.

   safety: good.

A third vaccine—*Flury vaccine*—is used for immunisation of dogs.

contains: virus attenuated by passage in chick embryos —LEP or low egg passage virus.

MARBURG VIRUS DISEASE

A severe disease which appeared in 1967 as a single outbreak initially involving laboratory workers in Marburg, Frankfurt and Belgrade. The patients had handled tissues from the same batch of African green monkeys. Later, there were other cases in contacts of the patients. The disease apparently originated in the monkeys which were carrying the virus.

Clinical Features

Clinically, the disease was a severe, febrile illness with a maculo-papular rash and haemorrhagic manifestations: other features were vomiting, diarrhoea, lymphadenopathy, hepatitis and signs of CNS involvement: the mortality rate was 23 per cent.

Virology

1. Very unusual virus particles, long, filamentous, with the ends often bent into a hook or a horseshoe shape: 665 nm by 100 nm.
2. RNA virus
3. Grows in various tissue cultures without CPE but with intra-cytoplasmic inclusions resembling Negri bodies
4. Pathogenic for guinea-pigs, monkeys and other laboratory animals.

Diagnosis

The disease has a very characteristic clinical picture. Confirmation of the virus aetiology in the original outbreak was obtained by isolating the virus in laboratory animals.

Isolation

Specimen: blood

Inoculate: guinea-pigs

Observe: for signs of febrile illness.

ARENOVIRUSES

LYMPHOCYTIC CHORIOMENINGITIS

Another disease contracted by man from animals: the virus causes widespread natural infection in mice and is excreted in the urine and faeces of infected mice: transmission to man appears to be a rare event.

The disease is of interest from an immunological point of view since mice are not uncommonly infected *in utero*: when this happens they have a generalised infection with high titres of virus in all tissues and organs: however the mice remain healthy and although they do not have antibody to the virus they are resistant to re-infection.

Clinical Features

The most important syndrome in man is aseptic meningitis: sometimes meningo-encephalitis is seen: the virus can also cause an influenza-like febrile illness.

Virus is spread to man by inhalation of dust or by contamination of food in infested houses.

Virology

1. Small virus—110 nm enveloped particles with the internal granules characteristic of arenoviruses.
2. RNA virus
3. Grows in the chick embryo and in monkey kidney and chick embryo cell tissue cultures
4. Pathogenic for mice and guinea-pigs.

Diagnosis

Serology

Complement fixation test.

Isolation

Specimen: CSF, blood

Inoculate: mice intra-cerebrally

Observe: for spasm of hind legs, tremors, convulsions and death.

LASSA FEVER

A serious febrile disease which was first reported in Lassa in Nigeria: the virus appears to be highly infectious and to spread by contact since some nurses who attended patients with the disease later developed—and died from—it.

Clinical Features

The illness is severe with marked weakness and malaise: sore throat with ulcers in the mouth and pharynx and cervical lymphadenopathy are characteristic features: myositis, myocarditis and pleural effusion are common and the blood count shows leucopenia: the case fatality rate is difficult to estimate in the small outbreaks described but several patients have died.

Virology

1. Arenovirus: about 110nm in diameter
2. RNA virus
3. Grows in tissue culture—in Vero cells (a monkey kidney cell line) with CPE
4. Non-pathogenic for mice
5. Slight antigenic relationship with lymphocytic choriomeningitis virus.

Diagnosis

Isolation

Specimens: blood, throat washings, urine, pleural fluid

Inoculate: Vero cells

Observe: for CPE of rounded granular cells with detachment of cells from glass
Type: by complement fixation test.

Serology

COMPLEMENT FIXATION TEST.

FURTHER READING

FRAME, J. D., BALDWIN, J. M., GOCKE, D. J. & TROUP, J. E. (1970). *Am. J. Trop. Med. & Hyg.* **19,** 670.
HABEL, K. (1967). Rabies: incidence and immunization in the United States. *Med. Clins N. Am.* **51,** 693.
JOHNSON, H. N. (1965). *Viral and Rickettsial Infections of Man,* 4th ed. ed. Horsfall, F. L. & Tamm, I. pp. 814-840. London: Pitman Medical.
KAPLAN, M. N. (1969). Epidemiology of rabies. *Nature,* **221,** 421.
SIEGERT, R. (1970). In *Modern Trends in Medical Virology,* **2,** ed. Heath, R. B. & Waterson, A. P., p. 204.

CHAPTER X

HERPESVIRUS DISEASES

HERPES SIMPLEX

HERPES SIMPLEX virus is widespread in human populations: its manifestations are protean in that it gives rise to many different kinds of disease: perhaps the most interesting property of this virus is its tendency to cause recurrent infections.

CLINICAL FEATURES

Herpes simplex infections in man are seen either as *primary* or *recurrent infections.*

Primary infections

The most common age for primary infection is from 2-4 years: many of these infections are symptomless: *the most common disease* associated with primary infection is *acute gingivo-stomatitis* (vesicles on the gums and buccal mucosa): *conjunctivitis* and *keratitis* are also seen as primary infections.

Herpes genitalis: an eruption of herpetic vesicles on the genitalia: herpes simplex virus may also cause *cervicitis*: in both cases infection is transmitted venereally: in genital herpes, the causal strains, known as type 2 herpes simplex, differ slightly both antigenically and biologically from the strains associated with oro-facial or neurological lesions (type 1 herpes simplex).

Neurological syndromes: *herpes simplex* is a neurotropic virus and has a tendency to spread to the CNS: it causes a severe form of *encephalitis—acute necrotising encephalitis* —which is characterised by the sudden onset of fever, mental confusion and headache: the main site of infection is the *temporal lobes* where there may be extensive *neuronal necrosis.*

Herpetic whitlow: a painful infection of the fingers: seen in nurses (especially if nursing patients with a tracheostomy from whom infected secretions may be widely dispersed): outbreaks amongst nurses have been described.

Neonatal infection: severe generalised infection in neonates is usually acquired from a primary genital infection in the mother so that no maternal antibody is present for protection: affected infants have jaundice, dyspnoea, hepatosplenomegaly, thrombocytopenic purpura and vesicular lesions on the skin: the mortality rate is high: the disease is usually due to the genital type 2 strain of herpes simplex.

Kaposi's varicelliform eruption: superinfection of eczema: commonly due either to herpes simplex virus or to vaccinia: the lesions bear a clinical resemblance to those of varicella: the disease is often severe.

Recurrent infections

The most common manifestation: is recurrent 'cold sores': these are vesicles which appear in a crop usually at muco-cutaneous junctions such as round the lips or nostrils: the vesicles progress to pustules with crust formation.

Between attacks the virus lies *latent* in the tissues of the host —probably in the sensory cells of the trigeminal nerve ganglion.

Virus becomes re-activated: by non-specific stimuli such as respiratory infections (*e.g.* common colds or bacterial pneumonia), fevers or sunlight: *spread* is via the sensory nerves to areas of skin supplied by the nerves.

Relapses are common despite the high levels of circulating antibody in patients with recurrent herpes sores: this is probably because the virus passes directly from cell to cell and is not released to exposure to antibody in the surrounding body fluids.

Other recurrent manifestations: *kerato-conjunctivitis*—a serious infection of the eye in which there is infection of the cornea which takes the form of a branching or *dendritic ulcer*: scarring is common and the disease tends to assume a chronic but progressive relapsing course: recurrent infection with herpes simplex may affect *mucous membrane or skin on any part of the body* including the genitalia.

Renal transplant patients under immunosuppressive therapy sometimes develop unusually severe recurrent cold sores: these take the form of extensive and spreading ulceration around nose and mouth which may extend into the oesophagus.

Epidemiology

Infection with herpes simplex is *widespread*: the incidence of antibody increases throughout childhood with a rise to around 70 per cent. at adolescence: the proportion of people with herpes antibody increases gradually thereafter: 97 per cent. of people aged 70 years or over have antibody to the virus. Many people with antibody have no history or sign of infection: this indicates that many infections with herpes simplex are *symptomless*. Herpes simplex virus has some of the characteristics of a *human commensal organism* in that although it may from time to time cause recurrent infections it usually remains latent in the cells of the host.

Virology

1. The main virus of the herpes group
2. Icosahedron particle, with 162 projecting hollow-cored capsomeres: many of the particles are surrounded by a loose envelope of material derived from the host cell (Fig. 8)
3. Medium size—120 nm
4. DNA virus
5. Sensitive to ether
6. Grows in various tissue cultures with characteristic CPE with ballooning and rounding of cells
7. Grows on chorio-allantoic membrane with production of tiny white pocks
8. Pathogenic for laboratory animals causing encephalitis.

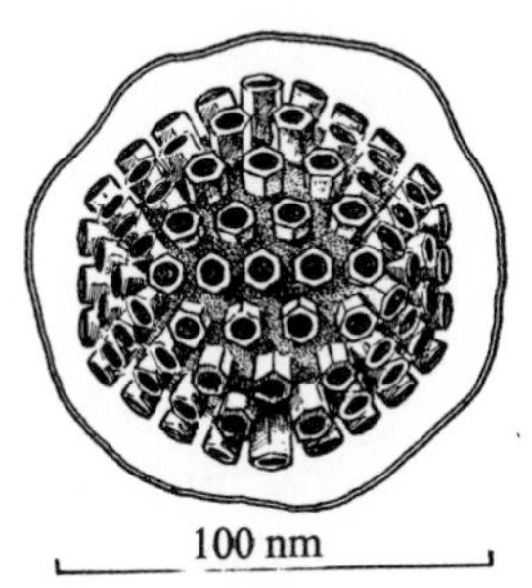

Herpes simplex virus

Fig. 8

Diagnosis

Isolation

Specimens: vesicle fluid, skin swab, saliva, conjunctival fluid, corneal scrapings, brain biopsy.

Inoculate: tissue cultures *e.g.* BHK21 (a hamster kidney cell line), human amnion or other cells.

Observe: for CPE of rounded cells.

Type: by neutralisation test with standard antiserum.

Serology

COMPLEMENT FIXATION TESTS: useful for diagnosing primary infections: difficult to interpret in recurrent infections because of high levels of existing antibody and because there may be no further rise in titre.

CHEMOTHERAPY

Idoxuridine is effective in the treatment of herpes simplex kerato-conjunctivitis and has also been used—apparently with some success—in the treatment of herpes simplex encephalitis (see p. 110).

VARICELLA-ZOSTER

Varicella (chickenpox) and zoster (shingles—but also sometimes called 'herpes zoster') are different diseases due to the same virus.

Varicella is the primary illness.

Zoster is a recurrent manifestation of infection.

VARICELLA

CLINICAL FEATURES

Varicella is a common childhood fever: there is a mild febrile illness with a characteristic vesicular rash: the vesicles appear in successive waves so that lesions of different age are present together: the vesicles (in which there are giant cells) develop into pustules.

The varicella rash has a close resemblance to that seen in smallpox which has been modified by vaccination.

Complications are rare: occasionally encephalitis or

haemorrhagic (fulminating) varicella: in adults pneumonia is a relatively common and serious complication and may be followed by permanent pulmonary calcification.

Prenatal varicella: if varicella is contracted late in pregnancy, the infant is sometimes born with generalised infection due to varicella-zoster virus.

Immunity: attack is followed by solid and long lasting immunity to *varicella.*

Epidemiology

Seasonal distribution: highest incidence is in autumn and winter.

Spread: via nose and mouth by droplet infection from infectious saliva: virus is also present in skin lesions.
Varicella is an epidemic contagious disease: it may be acquired by contact with cases either of varicella or of zoster.

ZOSTER

Mainly affects adults: clinically there is an eruption of *crops of painful vesicles* in areas of skin corresponding in distribution to one or more sensory nerves: the most commonly affected are the thoracic nerves and less commonly the cranial—including the ophthalmic—nerves.

Residual pain—which may be severe—often follows zoster in the elderly.

Neurological signs are sometimes seen—*e.g.* paralysis.

Virus is present in both the skin lesions and in the corresponding dorsal root ganglia.
The disease is *due to reactivation of virus* latent in dorsal root or cranial nerve ganglia following—and usually many years after—childhood varicella.

EPIDEMIOLOGY

Zoster—unlike varicella—is *not* acquired by contact with cases of either varicella or zoster—although it may give rise to cases of varicella in susceptible contacts.
Cases are *sporadic* and there is *no seasonal distribution.*

VIROLOGY

1. Member of herpes group of viruses: one serological type: in the electron microscope the particle is morphologically identical to that of herpes simplex
2. Rather large size, 150-200 nm
3. Grows in tissue cultures of human cells (*e.g.* human embryo lung or thyroid tissue cultures) with CPE but *the virus remains cell associated*: *i.e.* no free virus is released into the medium: this has greatly hampered investigation of the virus
4. The viruses of varicella and zoster have been shown to be identical in gel diffusion and fluorescent antibody tests.

DIAGNOSIS

Serology

COMPLEMENT FIXATION TESTS. Using infected human embryo lung cells as antigen.

Isolation. Rarely attempted.

CYTOMEGALOVIRUSES

Cytomegalovirus diseases are examples of '*opportunistic infections*', *i.e.* the viruses usually cause disease only when precipitating factors are present which lower the normal resistance of the host.
Cytomegaloviruses are the human equivalent of the 'salivary gland' viruses of rodents.

Symptomless and latent infections are common: about 50 per cent. of the adult population has antibody to the viruses but without developing any symptoms of disease.

There are two types of disease due to cytomegaloviruses:—

1. *Congenital infection*: neonates have a low resistance to infection and may develop severe *generalised infection* with cytomegaloviruses usually acquired *in utero* from mothers with symptomless infections in whom virus is excreted in urine or saliva.

   Signs and symptoms: affected infants have jaundice, hepatosplenomegaly, blood dyscrasias such as thrombocytopenia and haemolytic anaemia: the brain is usually involved causing microcephaly and motor disorders: surviving infants are usually mentally retarded: cytomegaloviruses are probably the cause of about 10 per cent. of cases of microcephaly.

   Affected organs: show characteristic enlarged cells (hence the prefix 'cytomegalo') with large intranuclear or 'owl's eye' inclusions: these are found mainly in the salivary glands, liver, lungs and kidneys.

2. *Postnatal infection*: *in children*, cytomegaloviruses cause *hepatitis* with enlargement of the liver and disturbance of liver function tests: jaundice may or may not be present.

   In adults, infection may take the form of an illness like *glandular fever* but with a negative Paul Bunnell reaction and usually no lymphadenopathy: there is fever, hepatitis and lymphocytosis with atypical lymphocytes in the peripheral blood: the syndrome is sometimes seen after transfusion with fresh unfrozen blood—presumably cytomegaloviruses, which may occasionally be present in the donor's blood, are normally inactivated by stora at 4°C.

Disseminated infection is also seen when *immunosu pressive therapy* or *severe debilitating disease,* such neoplasm, is present to lower the host's resistance. There a usually widespread lesions involving lungs as well as oth organs and tissues, *e.g.* adrenals, liver and alimentary trac this is a commonplace complication of renal transplantatio *severe retinitis* due to cytomegalovirus has been report in transplant patients.

VIROLOGY

1. Members of the herpes group of viruses: two serologic types: particles are morphologically identical to those herpes simplex
2. Grow in cultures of human fibroblast cells with CP and characteristic intranuclear 'owl's eye' inclusions.

DIAGNOSIS

Demonstration of typical intranuclear 'owl's eye' incl sion in cells of urinary sediment.

Serology

COMPLEMENT FIXATION TEST.

Isolation

Specimens: urine, throat swabs

Inoculate: human fibroblast cell cultures

Observe: for CPE which usually takes from 2-3 weeks appear.

"EB" OR EPSTEIN-BARR VIRUS

EB virus is a herpes virus which is associated wit cultures of Burkitt's lymphoma cells (Burkitt's lymphom is a common malignant tumour in African children): th virus is found in a variable proportion of cells in continuously-growing cultures established from the tumours: the cells grow in suspension and the virus does not produce CPE.

EB virus can be detected in the cells by *electron microscopy* —in which the particles are morphologically identical with those of herpes simplex—or by the *fluorescent antibody technique*—using labelled serum from a case of Burkitt's lymphoma.

Antibody to EB virus can also be detected by the fluorescent-antibody technique, *i.e.*, by testing for immuno-fluorescence in cultures of lymphoma cells containing the virus.

GLANDULAR FEVER

(Infectious Mononucleosis)

A disease usually mild but sometimes prolonged and debilitating which is most often seen in young adults. Characterised by lymphadenopathy, fever, sore throat with atypical lymphocytes in the blood: patients usually develop circulating haemagglutinin for sheep erythrocytes—known as the Paul-Bunnell reaction: the haemagglutinin usually disappears during convalescence: some degree of hepatitis is common: it is now known that *glandular fever is due to infection with EB virus.*

Antibodies to EB virus are relatively common in normal populations—indicating that infection with EB virus (presumably usually symptomless) is common: antibodies to EB virus are also present in the sera of 100 per cent. of Burkitt's lymphoma patients but the role of the virus in that disease is unknown (see p. 126).

Further Reading

Brain, R. T. (1956). The clinical vagaries of the herpes virus (Watson Smith lecture). *Br. med. J.* **1,** 1061.

Downie, A. W. (1959). Chickenpox and zoster. *Br. med. Bull.* **15,** 197.

Hope-Simpson, R. E. (1965). The nature of herpes zoster: a long-term study and a new hypothesis. *Proc. R. Soc. Med.* **58,** 9.

Niederman, J. C., McCollum, R. W., Henle, G. & Henle, W. (1968). Infectious mononucleosis. Clinical manifestations in relation to EB virus antibodies. *J. Am. med. Ass.* **203**, 205.

Stern, H. (1968). Isolation of cytomegalovirus and clinical manifestations of infection at different ages. *Br. med. J.* **1,** 665.

CHAPTER XI

MUMPS, MEASLES, RUBELLA

MUMPS

Clinical Features

Mumps is a childhood fever which is less common than measles: there is a relatively long incubation period of about 18-21 days.

Clinically: a febrile illness with inflammation of salivary glands causing characteristic swelling of parotid and submaxillary glands.

Neurological complications are also not uncommon: these usually take the form of aseptic meningitis or meningo-encephalitis: occasionally there is muscular weakness or paralysis. Neurological syndromes due to mumps virus are not accompanied by parotitis in 50 per cent. of cases.

Other complications: *orchitis, pancreatitis* and—very rarely—*oophoritis* and *thyroiditis* are seen in association with mumps: about 20 per cent. of adult males who contract mumps develop orchitis.

Immunity: an attack is followed by solid and long-lasting immunity: second attacks are very rare.

Mumps is a generalised infection by a virus with a predilection for the CNS (neurotropism) and for glandular tissue.

Epidemiology

Spread is by droplet infection with infectious saliva via the nose and mouth.

Seasonal distribution—the highest incidence is in the spring.

Age distribution: commonest in children aged from 5 to 15 years: but is not uncommon in young adults and outbreaks have been reported in recruit populations.

Infectiousness: lower than measles or chickenpox: as a result infection in childhood is not as common as with these diseases.

Importance is mainly due to the relative frequency of neurological complications especially when mumps infects adults: mumps is an important cause of meningitis.

Virology

1. Paramyxovirus, one serological type
2. RNA virus
3. Rather large in size—110-170 nm
4. Sensitive to ether
5. Haemagglutinates fowl erythrocytes
6. Grows in amniotic cavity of chick embryo and in monkey kidney and other tissue cultures with haemadsorption.

Diagnosis

Serology (widely used)

COMPLEMENT FIXATION TEST: Two antigens are used:—

1. 'S' or soluble antigen (the nucleoprotein core of the virus particle)
2. 'V' or viral antigen (found on the surface of the virus particle)

Antibody to 'S' antigen appears earlier but diminishes sooner than antibody to 'V' antigen: it is therefore a useful indication of recent infection

'V' antibody usually persists for years.

Isolation (Not so useful as serology)

Specimens: saliva—or CSF in neurological disease.

Inoculate: monkey kidney tissue cultures or amniotic cavity of chick embryo

Observe: *tissue cultures* for haemadsorption of fowl erythrocytes

chick embryo for appearance of haemagglutinin for fowl erythrocytes in amniotic fluid

Type virus: by inhibition of haemadsorption or haemagglutination with standard antiserum.

MEASLES

CLINICAL FEATURES

MEASLES is the most common of the childhood fevers: in uncomplicated cases it is a mild disease but complications are relatively frequent. For this reason, vaccines have been developed which are being used on an increasing scale.

Measles starts with prodromal respiratory symptoms such as nasal discharge and suffusion of the eyes.

The characteristic illness of measles follows: the main features are fever—which may be high—with a maculopapular rash lasting from two to five days.

Immunity following measles is life-long and second attacks are very rare.

Complications

The most common complications are *respiratory infections* which are seen in about 4 per cent. of patients; these include bronchitis, bronchiolitis, croup and bronchopneumonia; *otitis media* is also seen in about 2·5 per cent. of cases:

Before the advent of the antibiotics these infections were more frequent and were largely responsible for the mortality associated with measles.

Rarer complications are encephalitis and giant cell pneumonia:—

Encephalitis or post-infectious encephalomyelitis: a serious condition which follows measles in about one in every 1,000 cases: the mortality rate is about 50 per cent. and many of the survivors have residual neurological symptoms: encephalitis commonly presents with drowsiness, vomiting, headache and convulsions.

Subacute sclerosing panencephalitis: this rare disease is a chronic progressive degenerative neurological disease seen in children: at post mortem, there are numerous intranuclear inclusions seen throughout the brain: measles virus has been grown from the brain and the disease seems to be due to reactivation of measles virus long after recovering from natural measles.

Giant cell pneumonia: a rare complication, seen mainly in children with chronic debilitating diseases: it is due to direct invasion of the lungs by measles virus and is usually fatal.

EPIDEMIOLOGY

The attack rate in measles is high: virtually everybody in Britain under the age of 15 years has had the disease: in isolated communities where measles is not endemic and where the entire population is susceptible, attack rates of more than 99 per cent. have been recorded.

Spread is by inhalation of respiratory secretions from patients in the early stages of the disease.

Measles in Britain appears in widespread epidemics every second year; this is probably because in two years sufficient new susceptible hosts have been born into the community for the virus to become epidemic again: in non-epidemic years, measles is endemic but the number of cases is lower than in epidemic years.

In countries like Britain, where there is little poverty and malnutrition, measles is a mild disease with a low mortality rate.

In under-developed countries e.g. West Africa, measles is a severe disease and a serious cause of death in childhood.

Virology

1. Paramyxovirus, one serological type
2. RNA virus
3. Rather large size, 120-250 nm
4. Sensitive to ether
5. Haemagglutinates and haemolyses monkey erythrocytes
6. Grows in human amnion cells with syncytial CPE of multinucleated giant cells.

Diagnosis

Confirmation can be obtained by isolating the virus in human amnion tissue cultures or serologically by complement fixation test: but the disease has a characteristic clinical picture and this is rarely necessary.

Vaccines

A vaccine against measles has been developed because of the morbidity due to respiratory complications and because of the risk of encephalitis. Routine immunisation of young children is now officially recommended in Britain. The vaccine used is:—

Live attenuated virus vaccine

Contains: virus attenuated by passage in tissue cultures of chick embryo fibroblasts.

Administered: in one dose subcutaneously.

Protection: conferred is good with solid immunity which is apparently long-lasting.

Reactions: reactions such as fever and rash are fairly common but are milder than in natural measles.

Safety: vaccinated children are not infectious to others although virus multiplies in their bodies.

Normal Immunoglobulin

Normal immunoglobulin is derived from pooled human sera and therefore contains measles antibody: it has been used to confer passive immunity to infants and other unusually susceptible individuals who have been in contact with cases of measles.

RUBELLA

Rubella is a mild childhood fever but if infection is contracted in early pregnancy the virus may cause congenital abnormalities in the foetus.

Clinical Features

Rubella is a mild febrile illness with a macular rash which spreads down from the face and behind the ears: there is usually pharyngitis and enlargement of the cervical—and especially the posterior cervical—lymph glands.

Virus is commonly present in both blood and pharyngeal secretions: virus is excreted during the incubation period for up to seven days before the appearance of the rash.

Many infections are symptomless.

Complications are rare: these include encephalitis, thrombocytopenic purpura and synovitis (inflammation of tendon sheaths) which gives rise to painful joints.

EPIDEMIOLOGY

Rubella mainly attacks children under 15 years of age but many children reach adult life without being infected and infection in adults is not uncommon: about 15 per cent. of women of child-bearing age have not been infected and are therefore non-immune.

Infection is endemic in the community with epidemics every few years: the most extensive outbreak recorded was in the U.S.A. in 1964 when there were 1,800,000 cases.

The teratogenic properties of the virus were first discovered in Australia in 1941: it was noticed that an increase in the number of cases of congenital cataract had followed an epidemic of rubella: affected infants had been born to mothers with a history of rubella in early pregnancy and it was concluded that early maternal rubella can cause congenital defects in the offspring.

Congenital defects follow rubella only in the first 16 weeks of pregnancy; after that rubella does not damage the foetus.

The main defects are:—

- cataract
- nerve deafness
- cardiac abnormalities, *e.g.* patent ductus arteriosus, ventricular septal defect, pulmonary artery stenosis, Fallot's tetralogy

in addition affected infants have various disorders which, together with the defects, are known as *the rubella syndrome*: these are:—

- hepatosplenomegaly
- thrombocytopenic purpura
- low birth weight
- mental retardation

jaundice
anaemia
lesions in the metaphyses of the long bones.

The type and frequency of defect vary with the time of infection. Multiple severe defects are seen after rubella in the first six weeks of pregnancy.

The incidence of major defect after maternal rubella in the first three months of pregnancy has been found to be 16 per cent.: the comparable figure in a control group was 2·3 per cent.: maternal rubella was also associated with a higher proportion of abortions and stillbirths.

The total incidence of deafness increased to 19 per cent. when children exposed to rubella *in utero* were examined at the age of 3-5 years: the incidence of both deafness and defective vision further increased as the children grew up —probably due to easier recognition of these defects in older children.

Infants with the rubella syndrome have IgM antibody to rubella virus and therefore are immunologically competent (the maternal antibody which crosses the placenta is IgG antibody).

Antibody protects against re-infection and second attacks appear to be rare (some reported second attacks may have been due to other infections mis-diagnosed as rubella since rubella is not a particularly distinctive illness).

VIROLOGY

1. Unclassified virus, one serological type
2. RNA virus
3. Sensitive to ether
4. Haemagglutinates erythrocytes from day-old chicks
5. Grows in a rabbit kidney cell line—RK 13 with production of CPE and in other tissue cultures but without CPE.

Diagnosis

Laboratory diagnosis is usually reserved for pregnant women and for epidemiological research.

Serology

Haemagglutination-Inhibition Test: this is now widely used for confirmation of the diagnosis of rubella—usually in a pregnant woman or in suspected congenital rubella.

IgM antibody: recent infection with rubella virus can be diagnosed by the demonstration of IgM rubella antibody: this is because IgM antibody is only present for a short time after acute infection: IgM antibody is detected by fractionating serum on a sucrose gradient to separate IgM from IgG antibody: the fraction containing IgM antibodies is then tested by haemagglutination-inhibition for rubella-specific antibody: this technique is especially useful in pregnant women in whom only stationary titres of rubella antibody can be detected by standard tests: it can also be used to diagnose congenital rubella in infants.

Complement fixation test: but titres of antibody are lower and do not persist so long as haemagglutination-inhibiting antibody.

Vaccination

Live attenuated virus vaccine

Contains: virus attenuated by passage in tissue culture: virus is grown in either primary rabbit kidney cells or WI38 human embryo fibroblasts.

Administered: one dose subcutaneously.

Protection: good, immunity so far appears to be long-lasting.

Reactions: mild: sometimes slight fever and rash: mild arthralgia or joint pain is seen occasionally in adult females.

Viral excretion: a high proportion of vaccinees excrete virus from the nasopharynx but are apparently non-infectious to contacts.

Indications: schoolgirls; non-immune women of child-bearing age (who must avoid pregnancy for two months after vaccination).

Contra-indication: Pregnant women should not be given vaccine since it is not known whether or not the attenuated vaccine strain is teratogenic.

Normal immunoglobulin

Passive immunisation with normal immunoglobulin has no prophylactic effect in rubella.

Further Reading

British Medical Journal (1968). Report: Vaccination against measles. **2,** 449.

Dudgeon, J. A. (1967). In *Modern Trends in Medical Virology,* ed. Heath, R. B. & Waterson, A. P., **1,** pp. 111-140. London: Butterworths.

Manson, M. M., Logan, W. P. D. & Loy, R. M. (1960). *Reports on Public Health and Medical Subjects,* No. 101. London: H.M. Stationery Office.

Miller, D. L. (1964). Frequency of complications of measles, 1963. Report. *Br. med. J.* **2,** 75.

Reed, D., Brown, G., Merrick, R., Sever, J. & Feltz, E. (1967). A mumps epidemic on St. George Island, Alaska. *J. Am. med. Ass.* **199,** 967.

CHAPTER XII

SMALLPOX

SMALLPOX is one of the most severe viral diseases and has a considerable mortality rate. Control of the disease still presents many problems although effective means of preventing infection have been known since the end of the eighteenth century.

CLINICAL FEATURES

Smallpox is a systemic viral infection with a characteristic vesicular rash: the rash affects the face and extremities more than the trunk (centrifugal distribution): virus is present in respiratory secretions and in the skin lesions.

Incubation period: from contact to the onset of illness is on average 12 days.

First symptoms are of toxaemia, *i.e.* fever and malaise, and last for about four days.

Rash appears on the 16th day from contact: the earliest lesions are maculo-papules which rapidly progress to become vesicles and then to pustules with formation of crusts and scabs: the skin lesions all progress at the same time and do not appear in successive crops as they do in varicella.

There are two clinically distinct forms of smallpox:—

1. **Variola major (or classical smallpox)**

   The most important because the most severe form of the disease.

Toxaemia is profound with an *extensive rash* in which the lesions are deeply set within the skin.
The mortality rate is high—32 per cent. in unvaccinated subjects.
Facial scarring is seen in most survivors.

2. **Alastrim (or variola minor)**
A milder form of the disease.
Less toxaemia, less extensive rash with shallower or more superficial skin lesions than variola major.
Low mortality rate—0·25 per cent.
Facial scarring is usually less severe and seen in only 11 per cent. of convalescents.

EPIDEMIOLOGY

Smallpox was both endemic and epidemic in Britain during the seventeenth and eighteenth centuries: *Britain is now free from indigenous smallpox* but occasional outbreaks arise from the importation of infected cases from overseas: the risk of this has been greatly increased by air travel since the shorter travelling time has resulted in cases arriving in Britain within the incubation period.
The world incidence of smallpox is now declining fairly rapidly as a result of W.H.O. smallpox eradication programmes. However the disease is still *endemic* in the Far East and in some areas of Africa and South America: the outbreaks in England in 1962 were due to cases in immigrants arriving from Karachi where there was a severe epidemic of smallpox at the time.
Patients in whom the disease has been modified by vaccination are particularly dangerous because the disease may be *mistaken for varicella*: patients with fulminating infection may die before the rash develops and so constitute ' missed ' cases.

Patients are infectious from the 11th day or 12th day after contact—*i.e.* just before or at the onset of symptoms.

Maximum infectivity is during the first week of illness.

Source of infection: mainly virus shed from the respiratory tract: *respiratory virus* appears to have greater infectivity than virus shed in the scabs in the later stages of the disease.

Route of infection: by inhalation of virus either directly from the patient's respiratory secretions or from bedding and other articles contaminated by respiratory virus.

Smallpox does not have the high attack rate of measles or the capacity for rapid spread of influenza: under modern conditions of housing and sanitation it spreads only to a moderate extent mainly in people who have been in close contact with the infected patient.

Virology

The virus of variola major (variola virus) and that of alastrim belong to the pox group of viruses: this includes vaccinia virus (used for vaccination against smallpox) and cowpox virus together with various other animal pox-viruses.

The following properties are common to variola, alastrim, vaccinia and cowpox viruses:—

1. Large brick-shaped particles 200-300 nm (Fig. 9)
2. DNA viruses
3. Produce pocks on chorio-allantoic membrane of chick embryo that are characteristic for each virus
4. Grow in monkey kidney and other tissue cultures (with CPE with characteristic ' ballooning ' of the cells)
5. Haemagglutinate fowl erythrocytes

Diagnosis

In order that contacts be vaccinated as soon as possible after exposure to infection, it is essential to confirm the diagnosis in the laboratory as quickly as possible. The diseases most likely to be confused with smallpox (and especially smallpox modified by vaccination) are varicella, herpes simplex and possibly generalised vaccinia.

Specimens: scrapings from maculo-papules, vesicle fluid, crusts.

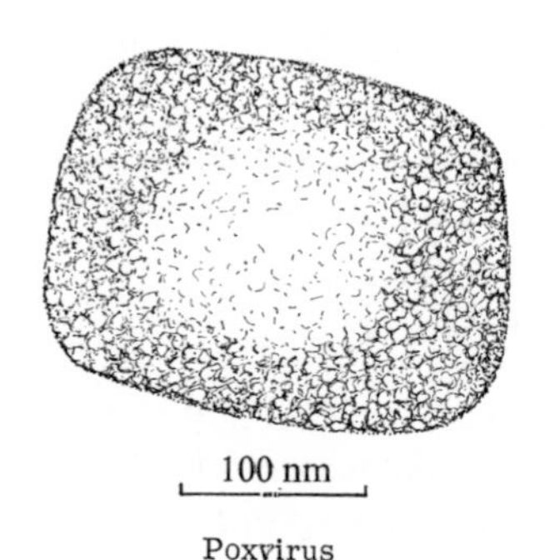

Poxvirus

Fig. 9

1. **Direct demonstration of virus:** poxviruses (with the exception of orf and paravaccinia—two animal poxviruses) have morphologically identical particles and so cannot be distinguished by this method: poxviruses can be demonstrated in two ways:—

   Electron microscopy: smears are examined for characteristic poxvirus particles. Time: 10 minutes.

   Stained smears: poxvirus particles are just large enough to be detected in the light microscope: Time: two hours.

2. **Detection of pox group viral antigen in skin lesions:**

These serological tests also detect only common pox group antigens:

Complement fixation test: material from the patient's lesions is used as antigen and tested for complement fixation with rabbit antivaccinia antiserum. Time: overnight.

Gel diffusion tests: material from skin is tested for lines of precipitation in agar with antivaccinia rabbit antiserum. Time: a few hours.

3. **Isolation of virus**

The only method of distinguishing between variola and vaccinia viruses.

Inoculate: chorio-allantoic membrane of chick embryo.

Observe: 2-3 days for characteristic pocks:—

variola major: small, white pocks (Fig. 10) which can also grow at 38·3 °C.
alastrim: small white pocks (identical with pocks of variola major but do not grow at 38·3 °C.)
vaccinia: large grey fluffy pocks with necrotic centres (Fig. 10)
herpes simplex: tiny white pocks smaller than those of variola
varicella: no pocks produced.

VACCINE

In 1798 *Edward Jenner* reported that artificial inoculation of cowpox protects against smallpox. Cowpox is a natural infection of cows which is sometimes transmitted to the hands of milkers from infected udders.

Vaccinia virus which is now used as smallpox vaccine differs in some respects from cowpox virus: however it is almost certainly derived from cowpox virus but has become

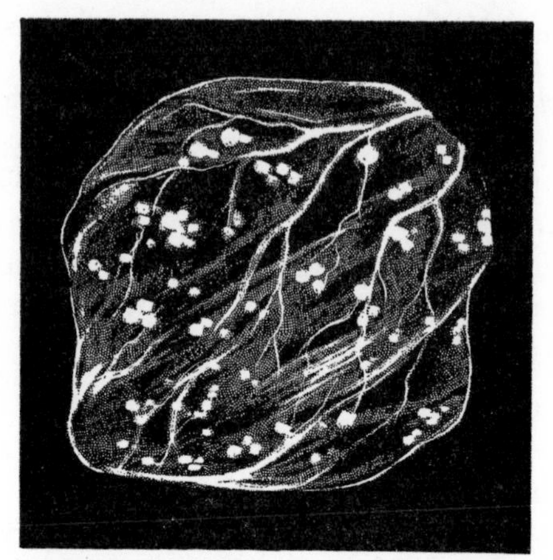

A: small white pocks produced by variola (smallpox) virus.

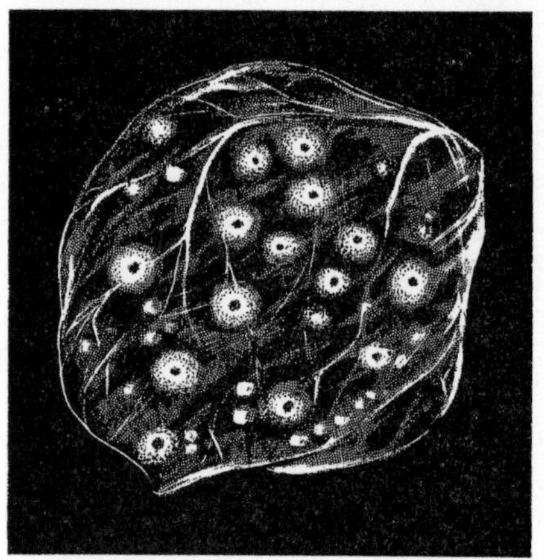

B: large grey fluffy pocks produced by vaccinia virus.

FIG. 10

Diagram of chorio-allantoic membrane of chick embryo inoculated with variola and vaccinia viruses.

altered during the frequent passage necessary to maintain it in earlier years.

There is a close immunological relationship between vaccinia and variola viruses: this explains why infection with vaccinia provides immunity against variola.

Smallpox vaccine today is prepared by inoculation with vaccinia virus of the shaved and scarified skin of the abdominal wall of sheep or calves: fluid (wrongly called 'lymph') is collected from the resulting vesicles and, after addition of glycerol to prevent bacterial contamination, is dispensed as the vaccine.

Vaccination: Vaccinia virus has a low infectivity for subcutaneous tissues and so is inoculated into the dermis: inoculation is carried out by making multiple light pressures with a Hagedorn needle through a drop of vaccine placed on the skin of the upper arm.

PRIMARY OR REVACCINATION VACCINIA: a vesicle appears at the 7th-8th day and the reaction reaches maximal intensity at the 12th day.

ACCELERATED REACTIONS: are also true reactions and are common in partially immune people: the vesicle appears at the 4th-5th day and the reaction reaches maximal intensity about the 7th day.

IMMEDIATE REACTIONS: are due to allergy to some constituent of the vaccine: sometimes an early vesicle forms but usually there is only a papule seen at the 2nd or 3rd day with some surrounding erythema.

Reactions should not be regarded as positive unless there are signs of vesiculation present at the 8th day after vaccination: *negative reactions must not be regarded as evidence of pre-existing immunity.*

PROTECTION CONFERRED: solid immunity against smallpox

lasts for about three years after vaccination: immunity wanes at a variable rate over the next 7-10 years.

Vaccination has a *strong and long-lasting protective effect against death from smallpox*: the mortality rate of variola major in unvaccinated patients is 32 per cent. compared to 10 per cent. in vaccinated patients but the *protective effect against an attack of smallpox is considerably weaker* and not so long-lasting.

Complications

There are two main kinds of complications after vaccination:—

1. ENCEPHALITIS: or post-infectious encephalomyelitis. Incidence about one per 100,000 vaccinations.
2. GENERALISED VACCINIA: seen mainly in infants and clinically divided into three types:—

   Mild generalised vaccinia: the most common complication in which the vaccine virus causes lesions outwith the vaccinated area: low mortality rate: incidence is about one per 25,000 vaccinations: sometimes *the lesions are numerous and severe*—especially if the patient is suffering from a condition which depresses the immune response: in these cases the mortality rate is high.

   Eczema vaccinatum: (or Kaposi's varicelliform eruption: which may also be due to herpes simplex virus see page 73): superinfection of eczema: in the majority of cases, infection is transmitted from vaccinated siblings who are dangerous sources of infection to a child in the family who has eczema: mortality rate about 25 per cent.

   Chronic progressive vaccinia or *vaccinia gangrenosa*: a very rare complication in which the vaccination gradually extends locally with severe and progressive tissue necrosis: some—but not all—cases have hypogammaglobulinaemia with an associated defect in cell-mediated immunity: the lack of cell-mediated immunity appears to prevent the normal tissue response which limits the extension of the vaccination reaction: usually fatal but thiosemicarbazone has given promising results in controlling the infection (see page 111).

Although complications are rare, the large number of vaccinations annually performed in Britain through the policy of routine vaccination of children in the second year of life resulted in a significant number of cases with serious complications: the policy of routine infant vaccination has therefore now been abandoned.

Pregnant women: should not be vaccinated because of the danger of severe foetal infection or *prenatal vaccinia*.

Control

Valid international certificates of vaccination are required for travellers entering Britain from endemic areas: if illness is suspected, quarantine can be enforced.

Outbreaks of smallpox are controlled by two main measures:

1. Prompt isolation of the case with disinfection of bedding etc.
2. Vaccination and surveillance of contacts.

Vaccination can only be successfully performed—and thus abort an attack of smallpox—in the early days of the incubation period: a significant advance has been the recent discovery that thiosemicarbazones prevent smallpox even if given late in the incubation period (see page 111).

OTHER POXVIRUS DISEASES

Molluscum contagiosum: A low grade infection in man characterised by reddish, waxy papules on the skin—most often seen in the axilla or on the trunk: it is a fairly common infection in children and is spread by close contact, *e.g.* at swimming baths: cultivation *in vitro* is doubtful but the lesions contain numerous poxvirus particles which can be seen in the electron microscope.

Orf or contagious pustular dermatitis: An infection of sheep and goats: occasionally transmitted to hands of animal workers causing chronic granulomatous lesions: characteristic oval particles in electron microscope with criss-cross surface banding.

Paravaccinia or pseudocowpox: The virus appears to be identical with orf virus: it causes lesions on udders of cows and is occasionally transmitted to hands of animal workers.

Further Reading

DIXON, C. W. (1962). *Smallpox*. London: Churchill.

CHAPTER XIII

VIRAL HEPATITIS

THERE are two forms of viral hepatitis:—

1. *Infectious hepatitis*: a naturally-occurring disease in which the principal route of infection is by person-to-person contact.
2. *Serum hepatitis*: a disease which is spread mainly by parenteral inoculation of infected blood or plasma or by the use of contaminated syringes.

CLINICAL FEATURES

Symptoms: jaundice, slight fever, nausea and vomiting: the urine is dark and the stools pale—characteristic features of obstructive jaundice. Serum hepatitis tends to be a more severe disease than infectious hepatitis.

Symptomless infection: common in infectious hepatitis: a proportion of cases of serum hepatitis are probably symptomless also (since infected blood is sometimes found to have come from people with no history of jaundice).

Prolonged viraemia: is seen in both diseases: virus may be present in the blood for some years after serum hepatitis.

The main differences between the two diseases are shown in Table VIII.

EPIDEMIOLOGY

Infectious Hepatitis

World-wide in distribution: endemic in most countries, epidemics appear from time to time: more common in rural than urban communities.

Age incidence: mainly affects children aged 5 to 15 years: but epidemics are seen in military recruit populations and children's institutions: food-borne outbreaks may involve adults predominantly.

TABLE VIII

INFECTIOUS AND SERUM HEPATITIS

	INFECTIOUS HEPATITIS	SERUM HEPATITIS
Incubation period	2-6 weeks	2-5 months
Route of infection	faecal-oral	mainly parenteral, some faecal-oral spread also
Australia antigen in blood	not usually	yes
Seasonal incidence	commonest in autumn and winter	none
Age incidence	mainly children	mainly adults
Mortality rate	0·1 - 0·2 per cent.	variable up to 30 per cent.

Primarily an alimentary infection: the site of entry and of primary multiplication of the virus is the alimentary tract: virus is excreted in the faeces.

Virus is present in blood and faeces during the acute phase of illness, but also during the incubation period: excretion in faeces usually persists for 3-4 weeks.

There are two main routes of infection:—

1. *Case-to-case spread* via the faecal-oral route: the most common route of spread of the disease: symptomless excretors may be an important—because undetected—source of infection.

2. *Via contaminated food and water*: numerous outbreaks have been described due to contamination of food-stuffs by a food-handler who is excreting virus or to pollution of water by infected sewage.

   The largest outbreak was in Delhi in 1955-56 where there were 29,000 cases following contamination of the main city water supply by sewage.

   Raw oysters and shellfish which have become contaminated by growing in sewage-polluted water have been responsible for several large outbreaks.

   Contaminated milk was the source of an outbreak involving 150 children in three country schools in Scotland: the attack rate in the pupils was 33 per cent.

Chimpanzees: may act as symptomless carriers of the virus and there have been outbreaks of infection in handlers of the animals.

Virology

It has not so far been possible to cultivate or demonstrate the virus of infectious hepatitis in the laboratory: experiments on the virus have therefore been carried out using human volunteers: these have shown that the virus has the following properties:—

1. resists 56° C. for 30 minutes
2. resistant to ether
3. serologically unrelated to virus of serum hepatitis.

Control

Passive immunisation: inoculation of normal immunoglobulin has a protective effect in preventing jaundice in people exposed to infectious hepatitis: there is no immunity for 2 weeks after inoculation but the immunity thereafter lasts for 4 to 6 months.

Serum Hepatitis

A disease seen mainly in patients who have received transfusions of blood or plasma from a donor with virus present in the blood: plasma is more likely to be infected because it is usually pooled from more than one donor.

Renal dialysis units: several extensive outbreaks of serum hepatitis have also been reported in the staff and in patients of dialysis units: infection is spread by blood transfusion to the patients and from them—as a result of contact with blood—to doctors, nurses and also to biochemistry technicians who handle infected serum samples: in some outbreaks, the mortality rate has been about 30 per cent., in others there have been no deaths: this suggests that there may be some variation in the virulence of the virus in different outbreaks.

Infected human serum: used in preparation of yellow fever vaccine gave rise to a large outbreak amongst American troops in the last war.

Syringes and needles contaminated with blood or serum have caused numerous outbreaks: a syringe which has been used for an injection is always contaminated with blood from the patient injected: syringes should therefore never be used for more than one patient (unless autoclaved between inoculations): outbreaks have been reported in V.D. clinics—where one syringe has been used for a series of injections of arsenic ('arsenic jaundice')—and in diabetic clinics.

Drug addicts: there is a high incidence of serum hepatitis amongst drug addicts who take drugs intravenously: this is because of the low hygienic standards of most addicts and because of the habit of using the same syringe amongst a group of addicts.

Track runners: in Sweden, where track running is a national sport, there has been a relatively high incidence amongst runners: infection is apparently transmitted by communal bathing with consequent contamination of skin abrasions acquired by running through bushes.

Tattooing: infection has been transmitted by tattooing.

Faecal-oral spread: there is evidence that serum hepatitis may occasionally be spread by the faecal-oral route: this is certainly a less common mode of spread than the parenteral route.

VIROLOGY

Australia antigen

Australia antigen (also known as hepatitis-associated or serum hepatitis antigen) is present in the serum of the majority of patients in the acute stage of serum hepatitis: in most patients, Australia antigen disappears on convalescence but sometimes it persists for long periods of time.

Carriers: some healthy people with no history of serum hepatitis are carriers of Australia antigen in their blood: carriage is much more common in people from Asia, Africa or Southern Europe than in people from Northern Europe or U.S.A.

In healthy blood donors in the West of Scotland, the incidence of Australia antigen is 1 in 800: all blood for transfusion should be screened for the presence of Australia antigen before use.

Antibody to hepatitis-associated antigen is rarer: it is occasionally present in the serum of patients who have had multiple transfusions.

Faeces and urine: recent reports indicate that hepatitis-associated antigen is present in faeces and urine as well as blood.

On electron microscopy: Australia antigen appears as ill-defined spherical particles 40 nm in diameter with smaller spherical and filamentous particles 20 nm in diameter: the larger particles probably represent the virus of serum hepatitis, the smaller particles being fragments of disrupted particles.

RNA: Australia antigen has been found to contain RNA —although only in small amounts.

RNA-dependent DNA polymerase: it has been reported that concentrated preparations containing particles of Australia antigen possess RNA-dependent DNA polymerase: this enzyme is also found in particles of RNA tumour viruses and visna virus (see pp. 117, 121).

Cultivation: the growth of Australia antigen in organ cultures of human embryo liver has been reported: replication was detected by the increase in the cultures of the titre of Australia antigen and in the number of particles found on electron microscopy.

Normal immunoglobulin: has no protective effect against serum hepatitis.

Diagnosis

Demonstration of Australia antigen

Specimens: serum (i) taken in the acute stage of serum hepatitis or (ii) for the detection of carriers

Tests:

COMPLEMENT FIXATION: the most sensitive test: patient's serum is tested against serum containing *antibody* to Australia antigen.

CROSSED-ELECTROPHORESIS: widely used, moderately sensitive: serum under test is migrated in an agar gel by electric current towards a known antibody preparation in a neighbouring well: the antibody moves towards the test serum by endosmosis due to the charge carried by the agar gel.

IMMUNODIFFUSION: the simplest test: the least sensitive

although sensitivity can be increased by 'topping up' the test serum and antibody wells after an hour or two.

ELECTRON MICROSCOPY: time-consuming but sensitive technique for demonstrating typical particles in specimens negative by other techniques.

Demonstration of antibody to Australia antigen

Tests are carried out by crossed electrophoresis or immunodiffusion by testing known Australia antigen positive serum against the test serum: evidence of past but not necessarily recent infection: rarely seen in acute phase or early convalescence of cases of serum hepatitis.

FURTHER READING

BRITISH MEDICAL BULLETIN (1972). *Viral Hepatitis,* **28,** No. 2.

GILES, J. P., MCCOLLUM, R. W., BERNDTSON, L. W., KRUGMAN, S. (1969). Viral hepatitis. Relation of Australia/SH antigen to the Willowbrook MS-2 strain. *New Engl. J. Med.* **281,** 119.

PICKLES, W. N. (1939). *Epidemiology in Country Practice*, p. 61. Bristol: Wright.

CHAPTER XIV

VIRUS INHIBITORS

VARIOUS substances inhibit viral replication *in vitro*: only a few are of clinical value but several have proved to be useful tools for investigating the mechanism of viral replication in cells.

Viruses are resistant to antibacterial antibiotics.

Idoxuridine

5 - iodo - 2′ deoxyuridine

Viruses inhibited: DNA viruses

Action: A halogenated nucleoside which is an analogue of thymidine: it becomes incorporated into developing viral DNA chains to produce malfunctioning molecules.

Uses:

1. *Treatment of herpes simplex keratoconjunctivitis* or *recurrent keratitis* (dendritic ulcer): applied locally as 0·1 per cent. solution: treated cases have a higher rate of cure but also more recurrences than untreated controls.
2. *Treatment of herpes simplex encephalitis*: administered by intravenous infusion but there is a danger of toxicity *e.g.* bone marrow depression: apparent benefit has been obtained in the cases so far treated but these are too few for the therapeutic effect of the drug to have been assessed.

Methisazone

1 - methylisatin 3 - thiosemicarbazone.

Viruses inhibited: Poxviruses.

Action: Inhibits a late stage in the virus growth cycle so that maturation or assembly of virus particles is prevented.

Uses: *Prophylaxis of smallpox*: reduces the incidence of smallpox in contacts of the disease even if given late in the incubation period: no therapeutic effect on the established disease: administered orally but vomiting is seen in up to 30 per cent. of those treated with the drug: the drug may not be lost because vomiting is usually delayed until 5-6 hours after dosage. *Treatment of complications of vaccination*: there is an apparent beneficial effect in eczema vaccinatum, chronic progressive vaccinia and other forms of severe generalised vaccinia.

Interferon

A protein released by cells *in vitro* and *in vivo* in response to virus infection.

Viruses inhibited: Most viruses are inhibited but RNA viruses are more susceptible than DNA viruses.

Action: Induces within cells the formation of *a second viral inhibitory protein* which acts on cell ribosome-virus RNA complexes preventing the translation of viral messenger RNA.

Species-Specific: Only human interferon acts on human cells: human interferon cannot at present be prepared in large quantities so other means have been investigated of inducing the human body to produce interferon as a prophylaxis against virus diseases.

Inducers: In addition to 'live' viruses, inactivated viruses, bacterial endotoxin and double-stranded RNA molecules induce interferon production in cells: the most powerful inducer is double-stranded RNA: synthetic polynucleotides such as polyinosinic-polycytidylic acid which have a double-stranded configuration are very active inducers and are under investigation for possible use as prophylactic agents.

Amantadine (and Rimantadine)

(1 - adamantanamine hydrochloride)

Viruses inhibited: Influenza A strains but not influenza B viruses, most parainfluenza viruses, adenoviruses and rhinoviruses.

Mode of action: The penetration of the viruses into cells is inhibited.

Uses: Under investigation for *prophylaxis of influenza*: orally administered: it reduces the incidence of naturally and artificially-induced infection with influenza A: side effects include amphetamine-like effects *e.g.* nervousness, insomnia and strange mental states.

Further Reading

Bauer, D. J. (1967). In *Modern Trends in Medical Virology*, ed. Heath, R. B. & Waterson, A. P., **1**, *pp*. 49-76. London: Butterworths.

Bauer, D. J., St. Vincent, L., Kempe, C. H. & Downie, A. W. (1963). Prophylactic treatment of smallpox contacts with N-methylisatin beta-thiosemicarbazone (compound 33T57, Marboran). *Lancet*, **2**, 494.

Patterson, A., et al. (1963). Controlled studies of IDU in the treatment of herpetic keratitis. *Trans. ophthal. Soc. U.K.* **83**, 583.

CHAPTER XV

SLOW VIRUSES

Slow viruses are a heterogeneous group of viruses which cause *chronic progressive degenerative diseases.* Several of these diseases involve the CNS. Slow viruses can *multiply for long periods of time* in the host animal without causing disease. In some—but not all—slow virus diseases, *production of antibody is minimal or absent.*

The main *importance and interest* of slow virus infections lies in the possibility that certain human diseases e.g. multiple sclerosis, amyotrophic lateral sclerosis, may have a similar cause.

The main features of slow virus infections are: —

1. *Long incubation period*: ranging from several months to many years
2. *Long, chronic, progressive course.*
3. *Severe and usually fatal disease.*

Slow Virus Diseases

Some of the principal slow viruses, together with their natural hosts and the diseases they produce are listed in Table IX.

Virology

Slow viruses are generally *difficult to isolate and assay* in the laboratory; this has hampered investigation into the diseases they cause. Visna and maedi are exceptions to this, and the causative viruses have been thoroughly investigated.

Little is known of the agents causing the other diseases. They resemble viruses in that they can be transmitted to

TABLE IX
SLOW VIRUS DISEASES

VIRUS	HOST SPECIES	PATHOLOGICAL FEATURES	DISEASE SYNDROME
Kuru	Man	Subacute cerebellar degeneration: status spongiosus	Postural instability; ataxia, tremor
Jakob-Creutzfeldt disease	Man	Subacute degeneration of brain and spinal cord with status spongiosus of cortex	Presenile dementia; ataxia, spasticity, involuntary movements
Mink encephalopathy	Mink	Subacute degeneration of cortex and brain stem: status spongiosus	Locomotor incoordination: debility, somnolence
Scrapie	Sheep	Subacute cerebellar degeneration	Ataxia, tremor, constant rubbing; susceptibility to infection is genetically determined
Visna	Sheep	Infiltration and proliferation of reticulo-endothelial cells in CNS; demyelination	Ataxic paresis, paraplegia
Maedi	Sheep	Gross proliferation of mesenchymal cells in lungs	Chronic progressive pneumonia with severe dyspnoea
Aleutian disease of mink	Mink	Plasmacytosis with hypergammaglobulinaemia	Wasting, anaemia; strong genetic predisposition to infection in mink homozygous for Aleutian colour gene

experimental animals and pass filters with a small pore diameter. The scrapie agent is almost certainly not a true virus, since it is resistant to ultra-violet irradiation at doses that would inactivate any nucleic acid present.

Below are brief descriptions of *visna, kuru* and *Jakob-Creutzfeldt disease.* Of the slow virus diseases, visna is probably the most fully investigated from a virological point of view. Kuru and Jakob-Creutzfeldt disease are described as the only examples of slow virus diseases which affect man.

VISNA

Visna is a chronic, progressive neurological disease of sheep. It first appeared in Icelandic sheep in 1935 following the importation from Germany 2 years earlier of the Karakul breed of sheep. Visna was eradicated from the sheep by a slaughter policy in 1951. It has been maintained in the laboratory since then by intracerebral inoculation of infected brain tissue into sheep.

CLINICAL FEATURES

The following are the main features of visna :—

1. *Long incubation period* ranging from a few months to several years.
2. *Slight paresis* is the first symptom: this usually affects the hind legs.
3. *Increasing paralysis* follows, leading to paraplegia and eventually to total paralysis and death.
4. *Virus is present* in blood, saliva and CSF during the incubation period in the first few weeks after inoculation of the virus. Once the disease is established, the virus is found in lungs, spleen and salivary glands as well as in the CNS.

5. *Neutralising antibody* appears early in the incubation period but, surprisingly, does not prevent virus multiplication in the tissues.

Virology

1. RNA virus
2. Medium size, 85 nm
3. Double-walled, roughly spherical particles with spikes projecting from the outer membrane
4. Does not haemagglutinate
5. Grows in cultures of sheep choroid plexus cells producing CPE of multinucleated stellate cells
6. Slow growth cycle in tissue culture with latent period of 22 hours and peak production of virus at 50 hours
7. Visna virus particles contain RNA-dependent DNA polymerase. This unusual enzyme transcribes DNA from RNA and is also found in RNA tumour viruses (see p. 121). The role of the enzyme in visna infection is unknown.

Kuru

Kuru is a fatal disease found only among the Foré-speaking people in New Guinea. It seems to have appeared about 60 years ago. The incidence increased up until the late 1950's when kuru was responsible for about half the deaths in the Foré-speaking people. The incidence of kuru declined rapidly in the early 1960's.

Clinical Features

1. *Kuru* is a native word meaning ‘ trembling with cold and fever ’.
2. *The first or ambulant stage* of the disease starts with unsteadiness in walking, postural instability, ataxia and

tremor: facial expressions are poorly controlled and speech becomes slurred and tremulous.

3. *The second or sedentary stage* is reached when the patient cannot walk without support, but can still sit upright unaided.
4. *In the tertiary stage the patient cannot sit upright* without clutching a stick for support: even a gentle push makes the patient lurch violently: the patient becomes progressively more paralysed and emaciated.
5. *Duration* of the disease averages one year but ranges from three months to two years.
6. *Death* is due to bulbar depression or intercurrent infection.
7. *Pathology*: neuronal degeneration in cerebellum with astrocytic hyperplasia, gliosus and status spongiosus; demyelination is minimal or absent.
8. *Sex incidence*: kuru is uncommon in adult males: most patients are women or children of both sexes.
9. *Cannibalism of dead relatives* is thought to have been responsible for the spread of kuru among the Foré people. Men do not usually take part in these cannibalistic feasts. The women and children eat the viscera and brains of relatives including those who have died of kuru. Since these tissues are often inadequately cooked the causal agent may be ingested in active form by those eating brain tissue.
10. *Cannibalism was generally stopped around 1957* and kuru is now declining in incidence: this lends support to the theory that the disease has been spread by cannibalism: on the assumption that kuru is spread in this way, the *incubation period* appears to be from 4 to 20 years.

Causal Agent

Transmission experiments: intracerebral inoculation of brain tissue from kuru victims into chimpanzees and other monkeys causes the animals to develop the symptoms of kuru after an incubation period of two years. After passage, the incubation period is shortened to about one year.

The reproduction of the disease in experimental animals is strong evidence that kuru is due to an infectious agent. However, attempts to cultivate the causal agent from both human and chimpanzee tissues in tissue cultures have been unsuccessful.

Experimental studies in chimpanzees have shown that the agent has the following properties:—

1. *Passes filters* of 100 nm pore diameter—indicating that it is in the size range of viruses.
2. *Present in infected brain tissue* to a titre of 10^6 infectious units per ml.
3. *Present in spleen, liver and kidney* of infected animals although the organs appear normal.
4. *Can be transmitted peripherally* (*i.e.* by combined intravenous, subcutaneous, intramuscular and intraperitoneal routes) as well as intracerebrally.
5. *No antibody* to the agent has been detected in either humans or chimpanzees with kuru.

Jakob-Creutzfeldt Disease

A rare progressive neurological disease characterized by a combination of presenile dementia with symptoms due to lesions in the spinal cord.

Clinical Features

1. *Prodromal stage*: the disease starts with tiredness, apathy and vague neurological symptoms.

2. *Second stage*: the patient develops ataxia, dysarthria and progressive spasticity of the limbs: this is associated with dementia and often involuntary movements such as myoclonic jerks or chorio-athetoid movements.
3. *The disease progresses steadily* until death—usually from about six months to two years after the onset by symptoms.
4. *Pathology*: diffuse atrophy with status spongiosus in the cerebral cortex: atrophy also in basal ganglia, cerebellum, substantia nigra and anterior horn cells.

Causal Agent

Transmission experiments: the disease is reproduced in chimpanzees and other monkeys after intracerebral inoculation of brain tissue from cases of the disease: the incubation period is from 11 to 14 months: the disease can also be transmitted peripherally (by combined intravenous, intraperitoneal and intramuscular routes).

Electron microscopy: virus-like particles have been observed in sections of brain from cases of the disease.

Further Reading

Gudnadottir, M. & Palsson, P. A. (1966). Host virus interaction in visna infected sheep. *J. Immunol.* **95**, 1116.

Hornabrook, R. W. & Moir, D. J. (1970). Kuru. Epidemiological trends. *Lancet*, **2**, 1175.

CHAPTER XVI

TUMOUR VIRUSES

MANY viruses have been isolated which cause cancer in animals. So far no virus has been shown to cause cancer in man.

The oncogenic or tumour-producing properties of a virus can be demonstrated in two ways:—

1. *inoculation of the virus causes tumour formation in experimental animals.*
2. *the virus transforms non-malignant cells in tissue culture into cells with the characteristics of malignant or cancerous cells*: *e.g.* rapid growth with frequent mitosis: or loss of normal contact inhibition so that cells in culture pile up on top of each other rather than remaining in the normal edge-to-edge orientation: transformed cells usually produce tumours on injection into experimental animals.

Table X lists the main animal tumour viruses.

RNA TUMOUR VIRUSES

RNA tumour viruses are generally more difficult to cultivate and to assay in the laboratory than DNA tumour viruses: the mechanism by which RNA tumour viruses produce the heritable change of malignancy—which presumably involves the cell DNA—has been difficult to understand. It has been shown that RNA tumour virus particles contain enzymes which replicate double-stranded virus-specific DNA off the virus RNA as template. This virus-specific

TABLE X

MAIN ANIMAL TUMOUR VIRUSES

VIRUS	NUCLEIC ACID	TUMOURS
Rous sarcoma virus	RNA	fibrosarcoma in fowls
Avian leucosis viruses	RNA	fowl leucosis (tumours of blood forming organs)
Mouse leukaemia viruses	RNA	Leukaemia in mice
Mouse sarcoma virus	RNA	fibrosarcoma in mice
Polyoma virus	DNA	multiple tumours of different kinds *e.g.* in parotid glands etc. in mice
Bittner virus	RNA	mammary cancer of mice
Shope papilloma virus	DNA	papillomas and carcinomas in rabbits
Adenovirus	DNA	sarcomas in hamsters
SV_{40} (simian virus 40)	DNA	sarcomas in hamsters
Human papilloma	DNA	benign papillomas or warts in man

DNA is then converted into double-stranded DNA. Presumably this DNA becomes integrated into the DNA of the cells causing the cells to become transformed into malignant cells.

1. *Rous sarcoma virus*: discovered by Peyton Rous in 1911 who found that the cell-free filtrate from fowl tumours produced sarcomas when injected into fowls: the virus can be assayed *in vitro* by the production of tumour-like foci due to transformation in monolayers of chick embryo fibroblasts.

Rous sarcoma virus can produce tumours in rabbits, mice, guinea-pigs, hamsters and monkeys in addition to fowls.

2. *Avian leucosis viruses*: infection with these viruses is widespread in poultry flocks—often without causing tumours: occasionally lymphomatosis—a kind of leukaemia in fowls—becomes epidemic and kills up to half the stock of poultry farms:

   In the natural state, leucosis viruses are transmitted 'vertically' *i.e.*, from hen to chick: chicks are often infected in the egg and contamination of eggs—including domestic hen eggs—is frequent: uninfected and non-immune chicks are susceptible to 'horizontal' transmission of infection from fowls which excrete the virus.

3. *Mouse leukaemia viruses*: these viruses produce leukaemia on inoculation into newborn mice: after passage through susceptible animals in the laboratory, their potency becomes increased and they can produce leukaemia in adult mice—and sometimes in rats and hamsters also.

   Laboratory mice vary in the incidence of naturally-occurring leukaemia: when low leukaemic mice are inoculated with mouse leukaemia virus, their offspring show a high incidence of leukaemia: the virus can therefore be transmitted vertically.

Mouse sarcoma virus: serologically related to Moloney mouse leukaemia virus: produces solid tumours and resembles Rous sarcoma virus in many properties.

4. *Mouse mammary cancer or Bittner virus*: Bittner agent —which is now known to be a virus—is transmitted in the milk of mother mice to their offspring: female offspring of infected mothers show a high incidence (92 per

cent.) of breast cancer: but if fostered by normal mothers the incidence of breast cancer in the offspring is 8 per cent.

Tumour development by Bittner virus depends on three different factors:—

(a) the presence of Bittner virus.
(b) hormonal influences: hormones are required to stimulate mammary tissue and render it susceptible to tumour development.
(c) genetic factors: strains of mice vary in their susceptibility to the induction of mammary cancer.

DNA Tumour Viruses

DNA tumour viruses are generally more difficult to culture from virus-induced tumours than the RNA tumour viruses: the viral origin of the tumour can usually be demonstrated by the presence of virus-specific antigens (which are not the same as the antigens of the virus particle) in the cells of the tumour: the viral DNA of some of the DNA tumour viruses has been shown to become integrated into the cellular DNA of transformed cells.

1. *Papilloma viruses*: cause non-malignant tumours or papillomas in man and animals, *e.g.* human warts: the virus of human warts has not so far been cultivated *in vitro*: sections of warts show numerous small icosahedral virus particles on electron microscopy.

   Shope papilloma virus is of unusual interest: it is the cause of papillomas in wild rabbits and is normally spread by insect vectors: it produces papillomas when inoculated into wild rabbits and in these tumours cancerous change is relatively rare.

   In domestic rabbits, Shope papilloma virus produces a higher incidence of papillomas and cancerous changes are far more often observed: virus cannot usually be cultured from the tumours which have undergone cancerous change.

2. *Polyoma virus*: polyoma virus is endemic in mouse colonies but is a very rare cause of naturally-occurring tumours in mice. The virus haemagglutinates guinea-pig erythrocytes and can be assayed by plaque formation in mouse embryo tissue cultures: it is therefore relatively easy to study in the laboratory: it transforms hamster cells in tissue culture into cells with the properties of malignant or cancer cells.
3. *Virus of progressive multifocal leucoencephalopathy*: a rare complication of debilitating disease particularly leukaemia or reticulosis: the main clinical signs are hemiparesis, dementia, impaired vision, dysphasia and hemianaesthesia: the disease is always fatal: a virus morphologically identical although serologically different from polyoma virus has been isolated from the brain of patients with the disease: it is not a tumour virus.
4. *SV_{40} or simian virus 40*: a not uncommon contaminant of monkey kidney tissue cultures: produces either no CPE or vacuolation of the cells: often present in monkey kidneys as a latent virus.

   SV_{40} causes tumours on injection into hamsters and transforms cells—including human cells—in tissue culture. The main importance of SV_{40} is that it is a highly oncogenic virus: it was a common contaminant of early batches of poliovaccine: as a result, thousands of young children were accidentally inoculated with the virus but apparently without ill-effect.
5. *Adenoviruses*: commonly cause respiratory infections in man: many types cause tumours on inoculation into

hamsters but types 12, 18 and 31 are the most highly oncogenic.

Adenovirus DNA can form '*hybrids*' with SV_{40} DNA: the nucleic acid of the hybrid contains fragments of the genomes of both viruses: hybrids are enclosed in protein coats specified by the adenovirus: cells transformed by the hybrids contain SV_{40}-specific antigens showing persistence of part of the SV_{40} genome.

Burkitt's Lymphoma

Burkitt's lymphoma is a highly malignant tumour which is common in African children: it is primarily a tumour of lymphoid tissue but the earliest manifestations of disease are large tumours of the jaw and, in girls, sometimes of the ovaries: it spreads rapidly with widespread metastases. Burkitt's lymphoma is very sensitive to cytotoxic drugs and excellent results with long-term remissions, and possibly even cures, have been described in patients treated with this form of chemotherapy.

There is a striking geographical distribution: the incidence of the tumour in Africa is almost completely confined to areas with altitude and minimum annual temperature and rainfall which correspond to areas in which disease-carrying insect vectors are found.

It has therefore been suggested that Burkitt's lymphoma may be due to a virus spread by an insect vector: however, there is as yet no definite evidence of a viral cause of this tumour—despite intensive investigation.

More recently, occasional cases have been reported outside Africa, *e.g.* in Western Europe and the U.S.A.

EB virus (p. 80) is of considerable interest: this virus is found in cultures of cells established from Burkitt's lymphoma: patients with Burkitt's lymphoma uniformly have antibody to the virus—detected by the fluorescent antibody technique—but so also do patients with glandular fever and a considerable proportion of healthy adults: it is therefore clear that infection with EB virus *per se* does not cause Burkitt's lymphoma: it has been suggested that the geographical distribution of the disease may be related to the fact that the areas where Burkitt's lymphoma is found are also those areas in which the population are virtually all heavily infected with *malaria.* In these circumstances the reticulo-endothelial system is heavily infiltrated with malarial parasites. It has been suggested that this may cause an abnormal response to infection with EB virus. As a result, EB virus, instead of producing symptomless infection or a benign proliferation of lymphoid tissue (as in glandular fever) becomes frankly oncogenic and causes cancerous change in lymphoid tissue (as in Burkitt's lymphoma).

Further Reading

Burkitt, D. (1969). Etiology of Burkitt's lymphoma—an alternative hypothesis to a vectored virus. *J. natn. Cancer Inst.* **42,** 19.

Fenner, F. (1968). *The Biology of Animal Viruses,* vol. 2, The Pathogenesis and Ecology of Viral Infections, pp. 641-700. London: Academic Press.

World Health Organization (1965). Viruses and cancer. *Tech. Rep. Ser. Wld Hlth Org.* **No. 295.**

CHAPTER XVII

BEDSONIA

THE group of related agents known as *bedsonia* which cause psittacosis, lymphogranuloma venereum and trachoma are not true viruses: they are placed between bacteria and viruses with respect to their properties and characteristics.

The main characteristics of this group of agents are:—

1. Large size (relative to viruses): 250-500 nm.
2. Visible under light microscope as blue particles with Castenada's stain or red particles with Machiavello's stain.
3. Intra-cellular replication with a complex growth cycle ending in a terminal stage of binary fission.
4. Contain both DNA and RNA.
5. Grow in yolk sac of chick embryo.
6. Sensitive to chloramphenicol, tetracycline and sulphonamides.

PSITTACOSIS (Ornithosis)

A disease transmitted from birds to man: *ornithosis* refers to the infection in birds in general: *psittacosis* refers to the infection in psittacine birds (parrots and budgerigars) in particular. Psittacosis in man takes the form of atypical pneumonia: this is usually a chronic infection and the lung lesions or opacities are slow to resolve.

EPIDEMIOLOGY

Ornithosis agent is widespread in wild and domestic birds: most infections in man are acquired from parrots and budgerigars but some are transmitted from other species of birds: *e.g.* epidemics among the Faroe Islanders have been traced to endemic infection in fulmar petrels.

Infected birds: many infections in birds are silent but some birds have diarrhoea, shivering, weakness, emaciation and purulent nasal discharge: the main lesions are in the liver and spleen.

Spread to man: is by inhalation of infected material from birds.

Occupational distribution: the disease in man is more common in those who work with birds, *e.g.* pet shop keepers, bird breeders, workers in poultry farms and people keeping birds as pets:

Britain: the disease is relatively rare in Britain.

Diagnosis

Serology

Complement fixation test: Antibody is demonstrated to a common group complement-fixing antigen shared by the agents of psittacosis, lymphogranuloma venereum and enzootic abortion of ewes (the latter is of low pathogenicity for man). The antigen used is the agent of enzootic abortion of ewes grown in the yolk sac of chick embryos.

Indirect complement fixation test: If testing sera from birds, antibody may react with the antigen but be unable to fix complement: avian sera are therefore tested for their ability to block or inhibit the complement-fixing properties of the antigen when it is subsequently tested with a known positive serum.

LYMPHOGRANULOMA VENEREUM

A venereal disease seen in the tropics (but occasionally in Britain also): males are mainly affected by the disease—females usually having symptomless infections.

The main symptoms: are swollen inguinal lymph nodes (buboes) due to sub-acute inflammation progressing to suppuration.

Diagnosis

1. Complement fixation test: to demonstrate antibody to the common group complement-fixing antigen.
2. Frei Test: a skin test to demonstrate delayed hypersensitivity to the agent: *intradermal inoculation* of a suspension of the agent grown in the yolk sac of chick embryos and inactivated by heat.

   Observe: for a nodule appearing at the site of inoculation within about four days: the nodule may persist for several weeks.

TRACHOMA AND INCLUSION CONJUNCTIVITIS

Trachoma

A widespread disease in tropical countries associated with poor sanitation and over-crowding: *highest incidence is in* children: the disease is a kerato-conjunctivitis which is often followed by corneal scarring: the disease is a *major cause of blindness* in tropical countries.

Spread: probably by contact or by contaminated fomites and flies.

Diagnosis

Direct demonstration of trachoma agent

Specimens: conjunctival scrapings stained by fluorescent antibody or with Giemsa or iodine.

Observe: for specific immunofluorescence or for characteristic cytoplasmic inclusions known as Halbertstaedter-von Prowazek bodies in conjunctival epithelial cells.

Inclusion Conjunctivitis (or inclusion blenorrhoea)

An acute *conjunctivitis* which usually clears up in three weeks: characterised by *inclusions* in the cells of the conjunctiva identical with those seen in trachoma.

Agent: similar, perhaps identical, to trachoma agent (sometimes known as TRIC or trachoma-inclusion conjunctivitis agent).

Natural habitat: the human genito-urinary tract: infection in females is probably associated with sub-clinical cervicitis: in males the agent may be associated with some cases of non-specific urethritis.

Diagnosis

Demonstration of specific immunofluorescence or typical inclusions in cells of conjunctival scrapings.

Further Reading

Meyer, K. F., Jawetz, E. & Thygeson, P. (1965). In *Viral and Rickettsial Infections of Man,* 4th ed. ed. Horsfall, F. L. & Tamm, I. pp. 1006-1058. London: Pitman.

Grist, N. R. & McLean, C. (1964). Infections by organisms of psittacosis lymphogranuloma venereum group in the West of Scotland. *Br. med. J.* **2,** 21.

CHAPTER XVIII

RICKETTSIAE

Rickettsiae are not true viruses: although they replicate only intra-cellularly, they contain both DNA and RNA: they should therefore be regarded as more like small gram-negative bacteria than viruses.

Rickettsiae cause various types of severe febrile disease which are *vector-borne* and are usually accompanied by a rash. The most important rickettsial disease is typhus.

Table XI lists the three main groups of rickettsial diseases.

TYPHUS

(Classical typhus fever—also known as gaol fever or famine fever.)

Clinical Features

Typhus: a severe, prostrating febrile illness with a characteristic '*mulberry*' rash: initially pink or red maculo-papules: the rash darkens to reddish-purple as the disease progresses: in severe cases, the rash may become petechial or haemorrhagic: respiration is rapid and photophobia is common. *Mental dullness* with interludes of delirium and leading to *stupor* is a characteristic feature: splenomegaly is often present and gangrene of the extremities is sometimes seen.

The mortality rate is about 20 per cent.

Causal organism: *Rickettsia prowazeki*.

Pathology

Typhus is mainly a disease of the capillaries of the skin and CNS: the endothelial cells lining capillaries are the

TABLE XI

RICKETTSIAL DISEASES

	Typhus Group		Spotted Fever Group	Tsutsugamushi Group
Disease	Typhus: Brill's disease (recurrent typhus)	Murine typhus	Rocky Mountain fever: other tickborne fevers	Tsutsugamushi fever (scrub typhus)
Causal organism	*R. prowazeki*	*R. mooseri*	*R. rickettsi*	*R. orientalis*
Vector	louse	flea	tick	mite
Host	man	rats	rodents rabbits dogs	? small rodents birds
Weil-Felix Reaction Patients' sera agglutinate *proteus* strains:—				
OX : 19	+	+	+*	−
OX : K	−	−	−	+
OX : 2	±	±	+*	−

* Variable.

principal cells affected: in the CNS characteristic 'typhus nodules' are found: these consist of perivascular accumulations of macrophages and lymphoid cells.

Weil-Felix Reaction: patients with typhus develop agglutinins in their serum for a strain of *proteus* known as OX19. The development of agglutinins for this and two other strains of *proteus* known as OXK and OX2 is characteristic of rickettsial infections: the reaction is rarely seen in other diseases: it may be due to an 'accidental' sharing of antigens by strains of both rickettsiae and *proteus* species: rickettsial infections may be partly distinguished by the differing patterns of agglutination for the three strains of *proteus*.

Agglutinins disappear on recovery but anamnestic responses (or non-specific rises in antibody levels during subsequent febrile illness) are common.

BRILL'S DISEASE

A mild form of typhus: due to reactivation of a latent infection following—and perhaps years after—a primary attack of classical typhus.

The Weil-Felix Reaction: usually negative.

EPIDEMIOLOGY

Typhus is an epidemic disease associated with conditions of *poverty, overcrowding and malnutrition.*

Epidemics have commonly attacked armies in the field. The disease broke out in Ireland during the potato famine in the nineteenth century and was widespread in concentration camps during the last war.

Vector: infection is spread by the body louse, *Pediculus corporis*: lice become infected with *R. prowazeki* which multiplies mainly in the alimentary tract of the louse: infected lice usually die in about two weeks.

Spread to man: *R. prowazeki* is transmitted to man by scratching of infected louse faeces into the skin surrounding the bite of the insect.

Bacteriology

The following properties are characteristic of rickettsiae in general.

1. Large size (relative to viruses) but small (relative to bacteria) cocco-bacilli approximately 300 nm in diameter.
2. Can be visualised under the light microscope: gram negative but best stained with Castenada's stain or Machiavello's stain, the organisms staining blue and red respectively.
3. Contain both DNA and RNA.
4. Replicate intra-cellularly in yolk sac of chick embryo and in mouse cell tissue cultures (demonstrate by staining with Castenada's or Machiavello's stain).
5. Rapidly killed by drying.
6. Sensitive to chloramphenicol and tetracycline.

Diagnosis

Usually by the Weil-Felix reaction

COMPLEMENT FIXATION TEST: can also be used.

Control

Vector control: *Anti-louse measures* are usually effective in cutting short an epidemic.

Therapy

Tetracycline or choloramphenicol are effective in treating the disease.

Vaccines

The two main vaccines are:—

1. *Cox's—or killed vaccine* prepared in yolk sac of chick embryos.
2. *Live vaccine*: contains the avirulent strain 'E' of *R. prowazeki.*

Q FEVER

Q or 'query' fever is a sporadic disease in Britain—and many other countries also: it is due to a rickettsia-like organism which differs in some properties from true rickettsiae: Q fever was first described as an epidemic of respiratory infection amongst slaughtermen in Queensland, Australia: infection is fairly widespread in cows and sheep in Britain but disease in man is relatively rare.

Causative organism: *Coxiella burneti.*

Clinical Features

The main forms of the disease in man are:—

1. *Non-specific fever* (*PUO*).
2. *Atypical or 'virus' pneumonia*: characterised by patchy consolidation: the disease tends to run a somewhat chronic course: severe headache is a characteristic symptom: mortality rate is very low.
3. *Subacute endocarditis*: seen in patients with damaged heart valves: the disease runs a progressive course and is nearly always fatal.

Symptomless infection: is common.

Epidemiology

Endemic in various animal species in many areas of the world *e.g.* sheep, cattle, goats, rodents, opossums, bandicoots and ticks.

C. burneti: is excreted in the milk of infected cows and the placentae of infected animals are very heavily contaminated.

Spread to man: mainly by ingestion of infected milk or by inhalation of contaminated dust or straw, possibly also by contact with faeces or placentae from infected animals: ticks act as vectors for animals but apparently seldom do so for man.

BACTERIOLOGY

C. burneti is similar to the rickettsiae in many properties but differs in being resistant to drying.

DIAGNOSIS

Serology

COMPLEMENT FIXATION TEST: with two different preparations of *C. burneti* as antigens

1. *Phase 1 antigen*: freshly isolated strains of *C. burneti* giving a poor reaction with acute or early sera but reacting well with sera from patients with long-standing chronic infection
2. *Phase 2 antigen*: strains of *C. burneti* after repeated passage in eggs: react well with acute or early sera as well as sera from long-standing infections.

In subacute endocarditis

DIRECT DEMONSTRATION of particles in stained smears of vegetative lesions on heart valves (taken at post-mortem).

INOCULATION *of guinea-pigs* with material from valvular lesions and spleen: after an interval guinea-pig sera are tested for antibodies to *C. burneti* by complement fixation test.

Therapy

Tetracycline and chloramphenicol are effective in treating Q fever.

Further Reading

Connolly, J. H. (1968). Q fever in Northern Ireland. *Br. med. J.* **1**, 547.

Snyder, J. C. (1965). In *Viral and Rickettsial Infections of Man*, 4th ed. ed., Horsfall, F. L. & Tamm, I. pp. 1059-1094. London: Pitman.

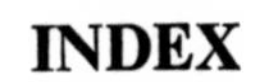
INDEX

INDEX

NOTES

Adenoviruses pharyngitis + conjunctivitis

Enteroviruses —

(i) polio group
(ii) Coxsackie group
(iii) echo group.

Respiratory syncytial virus (RS virus)
Bronchiolitis

EB virus - Glandular fever.

NOTES

NOTES

NOTES

NOTES

Printed by The Central Press (Aberdeen) Limited, Aberdeen